WHAT NURSES KNOW...
H E A D A C H E S

WHAT NURSES KNOW ...

HEADACHES

Wendy Cohan, RN

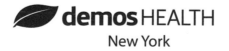

demos HEALTH

New York

Visit our website at www.demoshealth.com

ISBN: 978-1-936303-29-8

e-book ISBN: 978-1-935281-32-0

Acquisitions Editor: Noreen Henson
Compositor: Newgen Imaging
Printer: Hamilton Printing

Medical information provided by Demos Health, in the absence of a visit with a health care professional, must be considered as an educational service only. This book is not designed to replace a physician's independent judgment about the appropriateness or risks of a procedure or therapy for a given patient. Our purpose is to provide you with information that will help you make your own health care decisions.

The information and opinions provided here are believed to be accurate and sound, based on the best judgment available to the authors, editors, and publisher, but readers who fail to consult appropriate health authorities assume the risk of injuries. The publisher is not responsible for errors or omissions. The editors and publisher welcome any reader to report to the publisher any discrepancies or inaccuracies noticed.

Library of Congress Cataloging-in-Publication Data
Cohan, Wendy.
  What nurses know—headaches / Wendy Cohan.
    p. cm.—(What nurses know...)
  Includes bibliographical references and index.
  ISBN 978-1-936303-29-8
  1. Headache—Popular works. I. Title.
  RC392.C628 2013
  616.8'4913—dc23

                                                                    2012020145

Special discounts on bulk quantities of Demos Health books are available to corporations, professional associations, pharmaceutical companies, health care organizations, and other qualifying groups. For details, please contact:

Special Sales Department
Demos Medical Publishing, LLC
11 West 42nd Street, 15th Floor
New York, NY 10036
Phone: 800-532-8663 or 212-683-0072
Fax: 212-941-7842
E-mail: rsantana@demosmedpub.com

Made in the United States of America
12 13 14 15   5 4 3 2 1

About the Author

Wendy Cohan, RN, is a nurse, health educator, and health writer living in Portland, Oregon. She is the author of *The Better Bladder Book: A Holistic Approach to Healing Interstitial Cystitis & Chronic Pelvic Pain* (Hunter House, 2010). A practicing nurse for 18 years, Wendy also helps individuals take charge of their recovery from chronic health issues, including celiac disease, gluten intolerance, interstitial cystitis, and chronic pelvic pain (see www.WellBladder.com and www.glutenfreechoice.com). She is married to David F. Cohan, and is the proud mother of two grown sons. Her first book was *Gluten-Free Portland: Resource Guide.* Wendy also has lived with chronic headaches.

WHAT NURSES KNOW...

Nurses hold a critical role in modern healthcare that goes beyond their day-to-day duties. They share more information with patients than any other provider group, and are alongside patients twenty-four hours a day, seven days a week, offering understanding of complex health issues, holistic approaches to ailments, and advice for the patient that extends to the family. Nurses themselves are a powerful tool in the healing process.

What Nurses Know gives down-to-earth information, addresses consumers as equal partners in their care, and explains clearly what readers need to know and want to know to understand their condition and move forward with their lives.

Titles published in the series

What Nurses Know...PCOS
Karen Roush

What Nurses Know...Menopause
Karen Roush

What Nurses Know...Diabetes
Rita Girouard Mertig

What Nurses Know...Multiple Sclerosis
Carol Saunders

What Nurses Know...Gluten-Free Lifestyle
Sylvia Llewelyn Bower

What Nurses Know...Chronic Fatigue Syndrome
Lorraine Steefel

What Nurses Know...HIV and AIDS
Rose Farnan and Maithe Enriquez

What Nurses Know...PTSD
Mary Muscari

What Nurses Know... Headaches
Wendy Cohan

To my Mother, Helen Irene Sjoblom Jones, who soothed
my headaches with a gentle touch, a quiet voice,
and baby aspirin.

Contents

Foreword

As a nurse and headache sufferer, Wendy Cohan has a deep understanding of the impact and burden associated with having headaches.
What Nurses Know...Headaches is a one-stop shop for what you might
want to know about headaches: Are they a sign of a more serious illness, how might your headaches change over your lifetime, and what's
the process your doctor is likely to use to determine what type of headache you have. *What Nurses Know...Headaches* helps answer the many
questions people have about their headaches that may not have gotten answered in their usual healthcare appointments: Why do we get
headaches, what do headaches mean, and how can we minimize their
impact. Cohan addresses common and less common types of headache
and includes a chapter on the particularly difficult to treat chronic
migraine. Cohan also provides practical advice on treating headaches,
including a comprehensive review of effective alternative and non-
drug therapies. As a nurse, Cohan offers very practical advice, including a headache toolkit to keep on hand to help treat the unexpected

headache. *What Nurses Know...Headaches* is a must-have for anyone wondering why do I have headaches and what can I do about them.

Dawn A. Marcus, MD
Neurologist and Professor
Department of Anesthesiology
Pain Evaluation and Treatment Institute
University of Pittsburgh School of Medicine
Pittsburgh, PA

Preface

I am a big believer in the idea that "Knowledge is Power"—especially the power to take control of one's health. Teaching and "explaining things"—simply but accurately—is a passion of mine. Not everyone is in the medical field, but we all want and need to understand what is happening to cause our symptoms. But why did I choose to write about headaches? I wanted to provide clear answers for headache patients to questions such as *what* headaches mean, *why* they strike, and *how* we can help to alleviate, or prevent, problem headaches.

From an early age, headaches have been a part of my life, sometimes disappearing for years, only to reappear with alarming frequency or severity. Like many of you, my genetic background and the way my body responds to environmental influences simply makes me more susceptible to headaches. I've developed many coping methods over the years, which I share in this book. I was also inspired by the personal stories and suggested remedies that others so generously shared with me, and I am deeply grateful for their contributions to the book. Many of these stories are composites of several similar anecdotes, and I have also changed some names to protect personal privacy.

But, this isn't really a book of what it is like to *suffer* one of the dozens of different headaches discussed. It's a book about solutions, based on the latest research in neurology and exciting advances in the development of new headache medications. A revolution in understanding and treating headaches is underway.

In tackling this challenging topic, I've learned some things about myself too. Writing this book taught me to avoid pushing myself to the limit, as I have a tendency to do. I also learned the importance of having a backup plan when the usual headache treatments don't work. And, I can recognize the warning signs of a dangerous headache and take steps to have my symptoms evaluated by a doctor. There is an old saying that "nurses make the worst patients," in part because they have a tendency to avoid seeking help, even when they really need it. Throughout my life I have been "guilty as charged." But when I suffered my first sudden hemiplegic migraines after turning 50, I knew that I needed to seek help to rule out a more serious event. Knowing the warning signs comes naturally when you're a nurse, but this information is important to everyone, including *you.*

I love to write, and I hope that comes across in the flow of words across these pages. I love the thrill of research and pulling the pieces together to come to a true understanding of a complex subject. But most of all, I love to share knowledge, especially if it has the potential to help alleviate suffering in others. It is my way of "giving back."

Although I am trained in the hard sciences and have worked as a nurse for more than 18 years, I have come to deeply appreciate alternative healing methods and a holistic approach to whole-body wellness. I hope that my focus on headache *prevention*, through making positive changes in diet and lifestyle, helps people to move forward in their journey to better health and fewer headaches.

Introduction

As a nurse working on a busy medical unit, I learned a great deal about assessing and treating headaches of many types, occurring in both sexes and across the age spectrum. In a word, headaches are awful. There's an old English proverb that expresses the way many people feel about headaches: "When the head aches, all the body is worse."

Chronic headaches make the individuals who suffer from them miserable. Unfortunately, these disorders are very common in both men and women in all age groups. In fact, a staggering 45 million Americans have chronic headaches. Primary headaches, the most common category, include tension-type headaches, which affect nearly 78% of U.S. adults, and migraines, which affect roughly 12% of U.S. adults overall, but up to 17% of women. In an important meta-study (a review of multiple studies) in the United States, the prevalence of migraine headaches alone is equal to that of asthma and diabetes combined. The World Health Organization ranks headaches as one of the five most disabling conditions for women globally.

Diagnosis and treatment of headaches are major drivers of health-care costs, making up 20% of all outpatient visits to neurologists (doctors that diagnose and treat disorders of the brain, spinal cord, and nerves, as well as conditions involving pain or movement). The direct financial burden of caring for migraine headache patients in the United States is more than 12 billion dollars per year, yet nearly a third of migraine sufferers say they are not satisfied with their current treatment. It is estimated that the actual costs to society related to absenteeism, reduced productivity, and disability total an additional 12 billion dollars annually.

What can we do to reduce the frequency and severity of headaches and to prevent them from becoming chronic? Are preventive strategies the solution? Throughout this book, headache types are discussed in terms of symptoms, diagnosis, treatment, prevention, and risk factors. Some risk factors cannot be changed: family history of migraine, for example. But others, such as stress, diet, and the overuse of pain-relieving medications can be modified, through physician guidance, patient education, and support. Other preventive strategies include following specialized diets and using mind-body techniques such as deep relaxation, visualization, and biofeedback to help patients gain control over stress-related headaches. Nurses, including advanced practice nurses, are very experienced in patient education and can be your ally in many of these areas.

Living with frequent headaches deeply affects patients and has a very real impact on their families. I've seen a strong marriage greatly strained by a partner's chronic headaches before successful management was achieved. I've also witnessed a wonderful nurse and mother use her training and sensitivity to coach her migraine-prone son through relaxation and visualization, calming his headaches in as little as 15 minutes. And, I've personally experienced an intractable headache that failed to respond to a variety of expensive, and even invasive, treatments for nearly two full years, resolve completely with "Complementary Medicine." Headaches come in every shape and size, and for headache sufferers, success sometimes only follows the willingness to examine every possibility in terms of diagnosis, treatment, and perhaps especially, prevention.

One of my most memorable headache patients was a first-time mother hospitalized for a postpartum headache after the birth of her child. What a heart-wrenching experience it was for that poor young woman who wanted desperately to be home caring for her baby. Unfortunately, she was plagued with a completely incapacitating headache accompanied by sensitivity to light and sound, nausea, and severe pain. I stepped in after a social worker arrived to address the mother's "failure to bond" with her newborn. When the social worker began probing the patient about her feelings regarding being a parent, the patient understandably became very upset, yet her intense headache continued to overwhelm her ability to cope. I gave her an ice pack and a cold caffeinated drink and I phoned the doctor immediately for new orders. Less than an hour later, my patient was up, showered, dressed, and sitting on her bed packing, with hope in her smiling face. Her worried husband walked in with a cooing pastel bundle, and she reached for her baby immediately. There was nothing more on Earth she wanted than to be with her baby, but the headache had made it simply impossible. It was an important lesson for all of us in learning to listen to the patient, understand what they are trying to tell us, and believe their complaints of pain.

As a headache sufferer myself, I have great compassion for any headache patient in pain, and I've learned much of what I know about headaches from personal experience. I have had headaches all of my life. My head is my Achilles' heel, my weak spot, and my burden to bear. If only I knew then what I know now about headache triggers, headache prevention, and headache treatment, I would have had a much better chance at a headache-free childhood. I'll relate a little about my childhood summers to make this point clearer.

I grew up in Pennsylvania, where we travelled often to the lovely, rolling Laurel Mountains. Playing with my cousins and running through the fields and forests was fantastic! But even in my youthful enthusiasm, I quickly came to dread these trips because I was nearly always plagued with an extremely severe headache, sometimes lasting for days. No one in my family seemed to be able to figure out why.

Reflecting back, I know now that those trips to spend time with my grandmother and cousins, nearly three thousand feet above sea level in the heat of summer, were simply a "recipe for a headache"—especially for a headache-prone child. Those who experience frequent headaches (including those with migraine headache disorder) are often very sensitive to changes in daily routines, food intake, sleep patterns, and the physical environment, as well as to overexertion. Thus, the assault on my sensitive nervous system began early in the day. My grandmother stocked us up at breakfast with nitrite-laden breakfast meat, refreshed us in the afternoon with artificially sweetened cherry Kool-Aid and hotdogs or bologna sandwiches, then fed us canned ravioli for dinner. I never drank water, I never wore a hat, and I never took the time to lay down quietly when I felt a headache coming on. I wanted to keep up with my cousins—more streams to wade, more grape vines to swing on, more trees to climb! Finally, the headache would become too powerful to ignore, and my mother would be summoned to retrieve me. I would sob all the way home, cry myself to sleep, and usually wake up in my own bed, headache-free and ready for action.

Forty-some years later, I'm all grown up and an experienced nurse, too. I have taken charge of my own health, but I am still migraine-prone. The major difference is that I know my headache triggers and I do my best to avoid them. I am severely allergic to wheat and other gluten-containing grains, cane sugar, and dairy products. I can suffer terrible migraines related to food additives such as nitrites in processed meats and sulfites in preserved foods. I am careful to maintain good hydration and I have learned that drinking more fluids when travelling to higher elevations helps to moderate symptoms of altitude sickness, including mild to moderate headaches. I eat a well-balanced whole foods diet, exercise regularly, and try to avoid stress. I always wear a hat and sunglasses when I'm out for more than a quick walk. When I feel symptoms coming on, I take action immediately to prevent the development of an overwhelming headache, or worse, one that does not respond to my usual treatments. But, still, once in a while I get a really awful headache.

What are some other possible triggers? I've briefly mentioned that stress is an important factor, especially in the very common tension-type headaches. In women, hormones can play a big role, triggering headaches that tend to show up on a monthly basis through menopause, or, for other women, after menopause. Fatigue, overexertion, prolonged summer heat spells, withdrawal from caffeine and other addictive substances, or contracting a virus can all bring on a headache. I'll discuss many of these topics in the chapters that lie ahead, and throughout the book you'll learn the importance of avoiding dietary triggers.

As a nurse, health educator, health writer, and migraineur, I was honored to be asked to write *What Nurses Know...Headaches*. It has been an interesting and rewarding endeavor for me, and now I am pleased to share the results with you.

- Headache Basics and the four chapters that follow explain the causes of headache pain, help you to understand the difference between primary and secondary headaches, discuss risk factors and headache triggers, and provide tips for finding the right kind of physician and building your healthcare team. Also included here is a comprehensive review of Complementary and Alternative (CAM) therapies.
- Then we begin the discussion of primary headache types following the organization outlined by the International Headache Society. (Most familiar headaches are primary headaches.) In addition to information about risk factors, symptoms, diagnosis, and treatment of the most common causes of headaches, I'll share valuable detailed information about headaches in children and in women throughout the lifespan.
- Following a thorough discussion of the most common primary headache types, I provide important information about secondary headaches—those which are associated with other underlying illnesses and are not in themselves the primary health problem. In these chapters, you'll learn to recognize when a headache may be life threatening—and how to take action quickly. You'll also learn about the risk factors, symptoms, diagnosis, and treatment of headaches related to head trauma, brain tumors, infections, and inflammatory autoimmune diseases.
- Finally, we'll take a look at some future treatments on the horizon and I'll provide helpful information on coping measures and support strategies. These concluding chapters of the book also give you important information about tackling financial challenges and applying for social security disability.
- The Appendix, which follows the main body of the book, is a sample headache diary to provide you with a system for keeping track of your symptoms and triggers—a useful record to take with you to medical appointments.

- Finally, the book's glossary will enable you to understand "the language of headaches," which will help you to follow the information in research studies and to communicate effectively with your physician.

It is my hope that *What Nurses Know...Headaches* will become a useful, comprehensive resource for the millions of people who suffer frequent headaches, inspire patients to continue searching for answers, and help them to find talented and compassionate health care providers to guide their journeys to recovery. I am very thankful to the dozens of headache sufferers who shared their personal stories with us. And I wish you, the reader, the very best in health!

Acknowledgments

I would like to first recognize my husband David and my two sons, Bridger and Bryce, for having the patience and understanding to live comfortably with someone who suffers from headaches. It is not a walk in the park, for any of us. Those born to drum and wail on electric guitar should choose more accommodating parents! Bridger, thanks for helping with the references for the book. It was a big help, and probably not much fun.

I would like to thank the many health care professionals who have helped me with headache relief over the years, most especially neurologist Dale Margaret Carter, MD, Grant Dawson, DC, and physical therapist extraordinaire, Joe Keeney.

This book owes a debt to the compassionate, and *passionate*, work of Drs. Dawn Marcus, Christina Peterson, David Buchholz, Philip Bain, Stephen Silberstein, and many others. Keep up the good work— we headache patients deeply appreciate it.

Clair and Amber Davies's *The Trigger Point Therapy Workbook* was helpful when trying to visualize the anatomy of the head, neck, and shoulders and in explaining trigger points clearly. Cynthia Peterson's *The TNJ Healing Plan* was also a key to understanding how posture really contributes to headaches.

Also, thanks to writer and headache patient Paula Kamen, who helped put the experience of having an intractable headache in human perspective, with grace and humor. I thoroughly enjoyed *All In My Head,* which I found serendipitously (or as a gift of the universe) in an unlikely place, at the exact time I needed to read it!

Thank you to my good friend, Leslie Anderson, who put together the illustrations for the book, and listened to me work out my ideas and game plan for the book. You're a peach! Get ready to draw some more brains, my friend.

Thank you to the people who volunteered their time to read sections of the book and provide comments: Nadine Greszkowiak, RN, and Julie Glass, ND. You were under the wire, and you came through for me. I hope to return the favor some day—I mean it.

Thank you, wonderful state of Montana, once again, for giving me a quiet, undisturbed place to write, and write, and write. Once again, thank you to Laura and Bill and the rest of the Montana Boyd family for your awesome hospitality during my month amidst the berries and the bears. I'll never forget it, and hope to repeat it. (Say thanks to Steve, too.)

I am most thankful of all that I've been able to learn how to successfully manage my headaches, although life sometimes makes me take a refresher course. But that is how we learn.

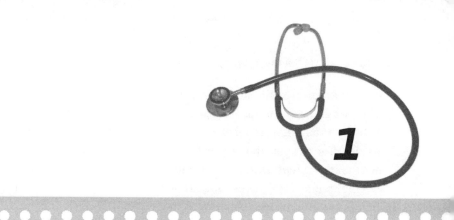

Headache Basics—Living With Problem Headaches

I have suffered from headaches most of my adult life. All of the conventional Doctors I have gone to told me my headaches were probably from stress and "just" tension headaches. Having raised children, especially through their teenage years, and working two jobs, I suppose I bought into it. Although, something told me it was more than stress. In the past five years I began having other symptoms, and the Doctors thought I had fibromyalgia, then Lupus, osteoporosis, arthritis and on and on. During this period the headaches and other aches and pains continued. I was at the point I would do whatever it took to avoid a headache, as anyone suffering from migraines or most any type of a headache would understand. The problem was, I did not know what to do... CHERYL

Headaches affect most of us at some point, perhaps because there are so many possible causes of headaches and because our highly developed nervous systems are sensitive to trauma, stress, diet, environmental influences, and overwhelming sensory stimulation. Learning to recognize, assess, and take effective action when a headache strikes is an important part of caring for our health—for all of us. But for people who suffer from frequent, chronic or severe headaches, it's *essential*. A mild to moderate headache, in isolation, is a normal physiological response to a fever, while a headache accompanied by vomiting, one-sided weakness or a stiff neck may be a sign of much more serious illness. Knowing the difference is both important and reassuring. This guide to headaches presents an overview of the major headache types, including tension-type headache, migraine headache, ice-pick headache, and cluster headache—and includes special chapters on headaches in women and children. This book teaches you to recognize typical symptoms and provides information on what you can expect in terms of diagnosis and treatment.

What We Know About Headaches

It isn't yet possible to know what triggers headaches in every patient— there are literally hundreds of causes of headaches. This is what makes headache medicine so interesting and also makes the treatment of headaches more of an art than a science, especially for patients with difficult-to-treat headaches, and the health care professionals who treat them.

Head pain, pressure, or inflammation can have a variety of causes. Inflammation plays a very important role in headaches, perhaps one of the most important. Inflammation may be related to the body's response to an infectious disease or a viral illness, and a popular migraine theory involves inflammation surrounding pain-sensitive blood vessels at the periphery of the brain and in the scalp. Dilation of these pain-sensitive blood vessels can be triggered by the ingestion of alcohol, foods containing histamines, or medications like nitroglycerine (used to treat some heart conditions). Headaches may also be related to musculoskeletal causes and problems in the muscles and joints of the neck or jaw, including temporomandibular joint disorders (TMJ, TMD). Nerve irritation is important in the case of neuralgias, including trigeminal neuralgia, postherpetic neuralgia (from shingles), and occipital neuralgia. (Neuralgia, often experienced as intense pain or burning along a specific nerve pathway, can be caused by nerve damage from systemic disease, inflammation, infection, or physical compression of a nerve due to musculoskeletal causes.) Even constant tension from a pony tail that is too tight or too heavy can irritate sensitive nerves at the back of the head, causing a headache. High blood pressure is often associated with a headache, although it may also be present with no recognizable symptoms. Significant or abrupt changes in blood pressure and changes in the pressure of cerebrospinal fluid cushioning the brain and spinal cord can be important causes of sudden, severe headache. But some of the most worrisome problems associated with headache, like brain tumors and aneurysms, aren't very common in comparison to the most likely causes of headaches. And frequently, headaches occur without a clearly identifiable reason, as is often the case with migraines, tension-type headaches, and cluster headaches.

Distinguishing Between "Primary" and "Secondary" Headaches

One thing that headache researchers and clinicians have agreed on is that there are two major classifications of headache types, and fortunately for the nonscientist, they are very easy to distinguish. Headaches that are the main problem, for which no other cause can be determined, are considered to be primary headaches. These include the most common headaches: tension-type headache, migraine headache, ice-pick headache, cluster headache, and several other headache types. In primary headaches, *which account for about 90% of all headaches*, the focus is on prevention and treatment. In addition to affecting the largest number of patients, primary headaches are the type most often seen by neurologists and they have the most significant economic impact on health care costs.

Primary headaches like migraine are thought to be triggered by a flood of inflammatory neurotransmitters in the brain, which may activate the trigeminal nerve and, ultimately, the adjacent pain-sensitive blood vessels and branches of the superficial temporal artery. This "neurophysiologic event" can account for many of the varied symptoms associated with many headaches, particularly migraines. The occipital nerve can also be involved in headaches, particularly headaches that begin at the back of the skull or in the neck, and some patients can suffer from a painful, chronic, nerve irritation known as occipital neuralgia.

Secondary headaches, in contrast, are associated with other health conditions, and treating the underlying health disorder can often lead to a resolution of the headache. About 10% of headaches are secondary headaches. A sinus headache is an example of one. Treat the sinus infection, then use preventive techniques to keep the sinuses clear, and frequent sinus headaches may cease to be an issue. In this case, it may be more important to view the beginning of a sinus headache as the body's warning sign that your sinuses are inflamed and need attention (the primary problem) than it is to treat the sinus headache (the secondary symptom) with medication. In fact, too-frequent use of headache relief medications can be the *cause* of some chronic headaches—and because the medication overuse is the primary problem, medication overuse headache (MOH) is also classified as a secondary headache type (Chapter 10—Chronic Daily Headache).

A few autoimmune disorders are associated with secondary headaches, and some metabolic disorders—including diabetes mellitus (DM), thyroid disorders, and kidney disease—may also include headaches as symptoms. The good news is that headaches related to these causes are often highly treatable by successfully managing the underlying health condition.

In more serious secondary headaches, conditions such as brain tumor, head trauma, or excess cerebrospinal fluid buildup can increase pressure against pain-sensitive tissues that lie outside the brain, primarily the meninges—the outer membrane enveloping the brain and spinal cord. The meninges are composed of three separate layers of protective membrane: the innermost pia meter, the arachnoid, and the outer dura mater. Meningeal irritation is suspected by some brain scientists to be the cause of many types of secondary headaches, including the painful and incapacitating headache of meningitis.

Doctors sometimes use a special acronym, SNOOP, to guide their assessment in distinguishing between primary and secondary headaches. SNOOP stands for: Systemic systems or secondary risk factors, Neurological symptoms or abnormal neurologic signs, Onset (sudden or abrupt), Older (new onset headaches in patients over age 50), and Previous history of headache (versus "first" or "different" headache).

Headache Theory Is Constantly Evolving

Most chronic headache patients suffer from one of the primary headache disorders, so let's take a look at important primary headache theories, past, present, and future. Traditional headache theory is constantly evolving, with the vasogenic theory holding sway since the late 1930s. This theory was especially applicable to migraines, including migraine with aura, in which a sensory disturbance precedes the onset of the headache. (Migraines will be described in Chapter 7.) The "vasogenic theory" was based on important clinical observations including the pulsating nature of migraine headache pain, its positive response to medications and vasoconstricting substances such as caffeine, and the ability of vasodilating substances such as nitrates to quickly trigger headache pain. Later research showed that levels of serotonin, a neurotransmitter, drop significantly during migraine attacks, and this discovery led to the development of an entirely new class of medications—the triptans. Imitrex (sumatriptan), introduced in 1993, was one of the earliest formulae and remains popular today.

The newer "neurogenic theory" holds that the brain itself generates the migraine, and the "threshold of susceptibility" of an individual to migraine triggers is intrinsic—probably due to genetic factors. This heightened sensitivity in an individual, in combination with environmental or other influences, influences the development of headache disorders. Great strides have recently been made in understanding the genetics of headaches, particularly migraine.

Innovations in diagnostic imaging technologies have also made it possible to observe changes in blood flow involved in migraines and related headache disorders. But neurogenic theory maintains that the vascular changes observed by researchers are a secondary effect, rather than the primary cause of the headache. This shift, from thinking of migraine in particular as a "vascular disorder," to understanding migraine as a distinct "neurological disorder," is important to the development of new treatments.

Since chronic headaches are the type most often seen by headache specialists and in headache clinics, there has been a great deal of interest in learning why episodic (infrequent separate event) headaches, which are not as difficult to treat, transform to become chronic problems, which are much harder to manage (see Chapter 10–Chronic Daily Headache). One explanation may be "central nervous system sensitization." Central sensitization results from increased activity in the central nervous system caused by an imbalance in the neurotransmitters that play a role in pain. These include serotonin, GABA, substance P, dopamine, and glutamate. It's a bit like having high-speed Internet along the affected nerve pathways, while the rest of us with "normal" pain processing have dial-up service. This process results in an increase in the number of, and responsiveness of, the body's pain receptors. Central sensitization can also cause pain messages to continue affecting the nervous system, resulting in lingering pain after damage has healed. For patients with chronic pain, the ultimate result of central nervous system hypersensitivity is a lowered pain threshold—meaning it takes less of a stimulus for the person to feel pain. Several studies have shown that stimulating pain receptors in the meninges lowers the threshold for previously nonpainful skin stimulation. For example, people with migraines may develop heightened sensitivity along the trigeminal nerve pathway, causing "cutaneous allodynia," the feeling of discomfort from simple, usually nonpainful, stimuli such as brushing the hair or touching the face. And although the popular headache medications called triptans are often very effective in eliminating migraine headache, they have a less powerful effect on allodynia. For patients with chronic pain and hypersensitivity, it may help to know that there is an explanation for their altered response to painful, and even nonpainful, stimuli.

No doubt headache theory will continue to evolve through advancements in scientific research with contributing support from clinical data. The newest information in headache research and its corresponding pharmaceutical development is located in Chapter 17–The Future of Headache Care.

What Are Our Headaches Trying to Tell Us?

Headaches send a powerful message. But what are they trying to tell us? Sometimes they're trying to tell us we're out of balance or pushing

What Nurses Know...

DOES THE BRAIN FEEL PAIN?

All pain from injuries and illnesses, and pain generated by the muscle, nerves, and tissues of head, neck, and shoulders, is recognized by the brain—but a peculiar fact is that the majority of the brain itself does not contain "nociceptors," or pain receptors. However, blood vessels that surround and permeate the brain tissue do have pain receptors, which is why the pain of a ruptured aneurysm, for example, is like no other head pain humans experience. The cranial and cervical nerves are also involved in headache pain.

ourselves too hard, or that we're not taking care of our physical being in a way that promotes homeostasis or equilibrium: drinking too little water, not eating properly, becoming sleep-deprived, or living life in the fast lane. We all need to nourish our bodies, minds, and spirits properly and get adequate sleep. As headache sufferers, we may want to try living in the shared commuter lane, with adequate support systems made up of family and friends.

In carrying out our jobs, we may be affected by factors such as poor posture, hunching over a computer all day, or eyestrain. On the other hand, making simple changes such as reading in adequate light and altering work routines to give our eyes a rest can help prevent headaches. Migraine sufferers are often very aware of their headache triggers and will make an effort to avoid the bright lights, inadequate sleep, or exposure to cigarette smoke that might trigger an attack. So can you.

There are some cases in which headaches are a sentinel, warning us that there is something wrong with the body; so casually treating them with painkillers without investigating the possible cause isn't really a good idea. It's like switching off the body's alarm system without searching for the source of the problem. For example, recurrent or severe headaches and occipital or high cervical neck pain should never be ignored or self-treated. These can be signs of serious, even malignant, diseases. I vividly remember a patient whose life was saved when, after spending dozens of fruitless sessions undergoing stretching, chiropractic manipulations, and special exercises, he insisted on seeing a highly regarded neurosurgeon for a thorough exam.

The patient's chiropractor was convinced that the headaches and vertigo were caused by a structural problem in the neck, when in actuality the patient had a large and dangerous tumor near his brain stem. He was very lucky to survive the lengthy and delicate surgery neurologically intact.

Sometimes, our headaches are so severe that they tell us we are in immediate danger and we need to take decisive action or depend on others to do so for us. A headache can be a warning sign of a cerebral aneurysm, which in a worst case scenario ruptures—leading to hemorrhagic stroke. In reality, most headaches are not caused by serious health problems, but it's important to be properly assessed, diagnosed, and treated for your headaches. As you'll learn in Chapter 13, sometimes a headache is not "just a headache."

What Nurses Know...

PAIN HAS A PURPOSE

Pain is a messenger that provides important information. At critical times, pain can even save your life by triggering your awareness of imminent or current tissue injury and motivating you to seek medical attention. And when you do, your accurate description of the nature and location of the pain helps doctors and nurses assess and treat injuries and illnesses. So removing all pain, by treating a head-injury patient with strong narcotics, for example, is dangerous—because it masks symptoms that may be necessary to make a lifesaving diagnosis and begin immediate treatment.

How Are Headaches Affecting Your Life?

Almost everyone gets a headache occasionally, but without successful treatment, the psychological toll of chronic pain can be a lifelong burden for chronic headache patients. Pain can be a very private thing and something we have difficulty sharing with others—even those close to us. Cindy McCain, wife of Senator and 2008 presidential candidate John McCain, did not discuss her frequent migraines with her husband for many years. Senator McCain was often away in Washington and she wanted to preserve their family time together without causing him additional worry. Writer Paula Kamen, author of *All in My Head*, also suffers from intense chronic headaches. She likens admitting your chronic pain to friends, family, and possibly coworkers to "coming out of the closet." Ultimately, being open and honest is the only way because there may come a time when you'll need the support and understanding of those people who are close to you. True friends will make allowances when you need to cancel or reschedule a social outing. If you're in a really bad headache period, both friends and family may even offer to help with shopping or childcare. Your coworkers may rally around you, helping to get you through this time with minimal stress or understanding your need to take time off. As a chronic headache sufferer myself, I'm well aware that we spend far too much time alone with our pain. I've learned that it's okay to let people in.

Beyond personal privacy, there are many other psychological aspects to headache pain which can create difficulties for patients. Three big ones are its hidden or invisible nature, its tendency to reoccur frequently, and its unpredictability. These are easy to see in real-life scenarios: "You don't look sick," or, "Another weekend down the drain—Why is it that I'm fine all week and then every Saturday starts with a migraine?" or, "I'm sorry—I know I said I'd drive carpool today, but it's just not safe for me to drive with the blurry vision I experience with my migraine, which I just happened to wake up with this morning."

Life with a severe chronic headache can make patients feel, and appear to be, unreliable. We all know we're capable of more, of better, than we are able to give during the pain and other symptoms of a severe headache. Sometimes strong feelings such as guilt, anger,

What Nurses Know...

JUST HOW MUCH DO HEADACHES IMPACT YOUR LIFE?

The Headache Impact Test, or HIT, combines scores from six questions to help quantify this issue. Take the test and find out how significantly headaches are impacting your life. The HIT test is available online at:
www.headachetest.com

and shame follow such events, but these emotions are a heavy burden to carry and are *not* helpful. It's understandable that you might become angry, at your headaches or yourself, but there certainly is no shame in being a person who gets headaches. Rather, there is courage in your ability to bear their unpredictable and bothersome effects on your life. Minnesota Senator and 2012 presidential candidate Michele Bachmann is a case in point. Known for having chronic migraines, Ms. Bachmann suffered criticism from those who felt that severe migraine headaches might hinder her ability to carry out the duties of the presidency. Her response was firm:

"I have prescription medication that I take whenever symptoms arise and they keep the migraines under control...Let me be abundantly clear—my ability to function effectively has never been impeded by migraines and will not affect my ability to serve as Commander in Chief."

Perhaps a little more media exposure is a good thing for those with migraines and other headache disorders.

Changing Attitudes toward Headache Patients

One of the most frustrating aspects of life with chronic headache pain is misconceptions on the part of health care providers. At times, we may suffer from age-old stereotypes about people who have migraines, who in the past have been thought of as driven, overly sensitive perfectionists. Writer Joan Didion recounted her experience in her famous essay on migraine headaches, *In Bed*.

> *"You don't look like a migraine personality," a doctor once said to me. "Your hair's messy. But I suppose you're a compulsive housekeeper."*

Doctor David Dodick, professor of neurology at the Mayo Clinic in Scottsdale, Arizona, has written,

> *"Medicine has long considered migraine and other headache disorders to be predominantly psychological afflictions of women, which is why many women have felt their symptoms weren't taken seriously."*

There simply isn't any truth to these age-old myths. In reviewing the International Headache Society (IHS) classifications for headaches, I found that even the world's leading specialists don't give much credence to headache as a psychological or psychiatric condition. Here are a few telling quotes:

> *"Overall, there is limited evidence supporting psychiatric causes of headache..." and "the vast majority of headaches that occur in association with psychiatric disorders are not causally related to them, but instead represent comorbidity (perhaps reflecting a common biological substrate)."*

The IHS classification goes on to explain that in the case of migraine, tension-type headache, and cluster headache, it can be particularly difficult to tell whether the pain is related to the psychiatric disorder or whether the headache is a primary headache that is occurring along with the disorder. Headache has been reported to occur frequently along with the following psychological disorders: major depression, dysthymic disorder, panic disorder, generalized anxiety, somatoform disorder, and adjustment disorder, but there is *not* a clear causal relationship.

We need to continue to work hard to overcome these stereotypes by educating patients and health care providers of all types. It is important to understand that primary headache disorders are treatable neurological conditions, and that headache patients deserve the same care and consideration as patients with any other neurological disorder. Fighting stereotypes and prejudice in health care should also include the awareness that all patients deserve excellence and equality in service, regardless of gender, race, creed, color, age, disability, and yes, even headache type.

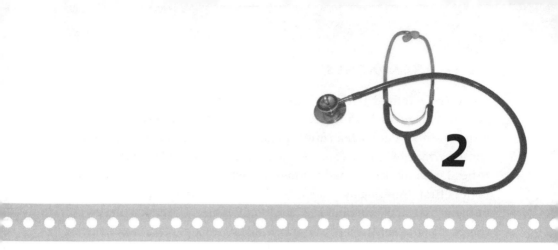

Understanding Risk Factors and Headache Triggers

I've experienced headaches over much of my adult life. Symptoms vary but they often seem to grow out of stiffness and pain in my neck. I sustained a moderate shoulder and neck injury on my left side when I was skiing over two decades ago. It seems like that side of my neck has never quite been the same. The stiffness seems to center in the scalene muscles, although I sometimes experience soreness in my upper trapezius. The pain in the neck can be severe and will migrate into the base of my skull. I call this type of headache "head on a stick." The pain is intense but unresponsive to both OTC and prescription pain killers and muscle relaxants. I get these headaches less often than I used to, maybe once a month now, so I just live with it.   DAN

There is a subtle difference between risk factors for headache and headache triggers. Risk factors cause people to be more vulnerable to a specific disorder such as migraine headache. Headache triggers, in contrast, may bring on a specific headache episode in someone prone to headaches, or occasionally in someone who is not. We'll discuss risk factors first, followed by headache triggers. In some cases, there may be some overlap. For example, smoking increases the risk of developing problem headaches, but simply inhaling second-hand smoke can also trigger a headache in a susceptible nonsmoker.

Risk Factors

The risk factors for developing problem headaches are many and varied, and include the following:

- Family history
- Stress
- Poor posture
- Low vitamin D level
- Obesity
- Smoking

Some risk factors, like obesity and low vitamin D level, can often be modified to reduce risk, while others, like one's genetics, cannot. Although some modifiable risk factors may be overlooked by headache sufferers, making appropriate lifestyle changes is something only each of us alone can do.

YOUR FAMILY HISTORY

We inherit genes from both of our parents, and if those genes include a susceptibility or vulnerability to headaches, chances are that we're likely to develop headaches at some point in life. This may be especially true in headache disorders such as migraine, abdominal migraine in children, and cluster headache. Family history is one risk factor we cannot change. But many other risk factors presented in this chapter can be modified, and in doing so, will help to decrease your overall chances for developing problem headaches.

STRESS

Stress has a huge psychological impact in all of us, and most health practitioners are well aware that stress can also cause physical symptoms, including contributing significantly to headaches. In a large survey on global human health, nearly half of Americans reported that stress and chronic worrying prevented them from getting adequate sleep and affected their mental health! Take an honest look at your level of stress, as well as your mood, on a daily basis: Are you chronically unhappy, irritable, or angry? Ask yourself some important questions to identify whether stress might be a significant problem in your life and whether it might also be part of your headache picture.

- Do you carry tension in your neck and your shoulders?
- Do you clench your teeth and jaws so hard that they ache? Do you grind your teeth at night?
- Do you sometimes feel tightness in your chest, making it difficult to take a deep breath?

Physical therapists who treat headache patients report that all of these signs of chronic stress are common. Take a yoga or meditation class from an experienced instructor and explore some of these areas of health. Develop greater mind-body awareness and master simple techniques you can use to decrease your level of stress and anxiety, including: deep breathing, relaxation, meditation, and yoga or chi gong. You might also begin to make important changes in your life that actually decrease your stress level and your headache frequency, including giving up stressful relationships and unproductive activities, switching jobs, or even re-inventing your career.

POOR POSTURE

Are you aware that problems with your musculoskeletal system can contribute to head, neck, and shoulder pain? Musculoskeletal dysfunction involving the head, neck, and spine is an important factor in generating headaches, as you can see in Dan's story at the beginning of this chapter. There is a specific category of headache called cervicogenic headache—one generated by the neck. Certain movements (or restrictions) of the cervical spine, or neck, can refer pain to the head via the occipital and suboccipital nerves.

A new study published in the journal *Spine* investigated the connection between the muscles of the suboccipital triangle (the rectus capitus muscle group) and cervicogenic headache, which is often experienced as tension headache. These muscles and the upper trapezius muscles between the shoulders and the neck are strained when the head is allowed to droop forward—known as "head forward posture." (See Figure 2.1) This position leaves the heavy head unsupported and tremendously strains the neck muscles. Tension headaches are common in people with chronic head-forward posture because these muscles ultimately connect to the dura mater, the outermost layer of the meninges covering the brain and the spinal cord, and constant muscle tension can result in irritation of the occipital and/or meningeal nerves. Take a closer look at your musculoskeletal system preferably with the help of a professional physical therapist and consider the following:

- Do you sit hunched over your desk or computer keyboard?
- Do you slouch at night on the couch while you watch TV?

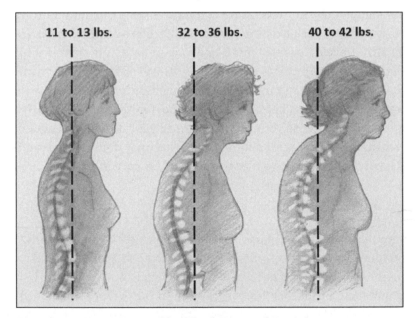

Figure 2.1 Force Exerted by Head-Forward Position

- Is your body moving well and easily, or are there areas of restriction?
- Is your body reacting to the limitations (desk job), or challenges (heavy construction), of your work routine?

Head-forward posture strains the muscles in the upper back and neck, and forces the muscles that keep the chin raised to stay contracted. This compresses nerves which lead to tension headaches at the base of the skull. A head forward posture makes the neck and shoulders feel as if they are carrying an additional 20-30 lb.

Work with a chiropractor or physical therapist on treatment, exercises, and preventive techniques for cervicogenic headache. Here is a great tip that my physical therapist gave me: *"Raise the sternum, and the head and neck will follow naturally."* Try it—it works. You may also find that, over a long period of time, a shaped foam orthopedic neck pillow from your local bed and bath store may be effective in maintaining proper alignment of the upper spine and neck—helping to prevent this type of headache. I would never travel without mine.

VITAMIN D DEFICIENCY

Vitamin D is actually a hormone made by the body when skin is exposed to ultraviolet B radiation from sunlight. It has long been known to

What Nurses Know...

Maintaining flexibility of the muscles and joints of the neck is important in preventing and helping to treat cervicogenic headache. A good exercise to practice several times a day is to slowly rotate the head as if your nose is drawing a circle or spiral in the air. To avoid dizziness, keep your eyes open and moving in the same direction as you rotate your head. More helpful exercises for people with tense neck and shoulder muscles can be found in Cynthia Peterson's excellent book, The TMJ Healing Plan.

play a role in calcium absorption but has more recently been found to play other important roles. It is now more common for doctors to test patients for vitamin D levels when doing routine blood-work. Research published in 2008 has shown that 41.8% of patients with chronic migraine were deficient in 25-hydroxyvitamin D and people who had suffered the longest from chronic migraine were more likely to be vitamin D-deficient. This is not good news, because low vitamin-D status also increases the risk for cardiovascular disease, chronic pain syndromes, and depression. A large study published in 2010 also identified low vitamin D levels in patients who suffered from migraine and other primary headaches, prompting researchers to state that "vitamin D may play some yet unknown role in multiple painful chronic conditions and possibly headache and migraine disorders." People in this study who suffered from chronic pain or migraine headache had levels, on average, about half of the optimum vitamin D level.

Vitamin D insufficiency and deficiency are common in the elderly, dark-skinned individuals, people who don't get enough sun, people with fat malabsorption syndromes such as celiac disease, obese individuals, and people with limited diets. Women and all persons over age 49 are more likely to be low in vitamin D. Vitamin D has anti-inflammatory and pain-relieving properties, and a few case studies have shown that supplementing with vitamin D had a positive effect on reducing both chronic migraine headache and chronic tension-type headache. More studies are needed before appropriate vitamin D supplementation becomes accepted practice in headache prevention and treatment.

The good news is that it is fairly easy to correct low vitamin D levels with the guidance of a knowledgeable physician. Your body

What Nurses Know...

It is also interesting to note that more people suffer from migraine and tension-type headaches in geographic regions more distant from the equator and during the low-sunlight winter months.

can begin producing vitamin D after exposing skin to direct sunlight for as little as 15 minutes a day. Vitamin D is also available over the counter as an inexpensive and well-tolerated supplement, but you should consult with a doctor on your vitamin D level before you start. Vitamin D is a fat-soluble vitamin and can be toxic if taken in excess, but its general benefits are so significant that the suggested dosage has been revised upward from previous recommendations. Some food sources of vitamin D include the following:

- Fatty ocean fish (salmon, tuna, mackerel, sardines, and cod liver oil)
- Egg yolks
- Fortified milk
- Liver
- Vitamin D-fortified dairy products

But it may not be possible to take in sufficient vitamin D from diet alone. It is also important to be aware that certain medications including anticonvulsants and some cholesterol-reducing drugs can interfere with vitamin D absorption. People with health conditions that result in excess blood calcium levels should not take vitamin D without consulting a physician.

OBESITY

One in three American adults is obese, which is defined as having excess body fat as measured by a body mass index (BMI) equal to or greater than 30 kg/m². We've all heard about the dire consequences of obesity, including skyrocketing rates of type 2 diabetes, heart disease, obstructive sleep apnea, and other preventable illnesses, but this condition is also linked to an increased risk for chronic headaches. A landmark study was conducted by pain specialist Dr. Dawn Marcus, who had previously noted that proinflammatory chemicals known as cytokines were implicated in migraine headache. She found that increased levels of cytokines were also found in people who were obese. Dr. Marcus examined 61 headache patients to further study the possible association between obesity and migraine headache. This small pilot study showed a relationship between obesity and test scores ranking pain severity, psychological distress, and quality of life. Other larger studies have shown that obesity roughly doubled the risk of developing chronic daily headache and was also identified as a risk factor in episodic migraine headache. Dr. Christina Peterson, a headache specialist in Portland, Oregon, wrote that "We do not yet know whether losing weight will reduce the frequency and severity of headaches...some headache specialists...suspect that the same risk factors that contribute to obesity also contribute to headache." And she points out that so far studies have shown that headache patients who are obese are just as responsive to treatment as patients who are not overweight.

SMOKING

Smoking is a very important factor that may contribute to headaches and it is one that we can control, although many ex-smokers would agree that it isn't easy to quit the habit. Several important studies have linked smoking with increased risk of migraine. A recent survey of over 1,000 Detroit residents revealed that migraine sufferers were nearly twice as likely to smoke as those who don't get migraines. Other studies have shown that smokers tended to have more severe headache symptoms and that smoking increases the risk of headaches in teens.

The Michigan Headache Institute offers the following possible mechanisms for the influence of smoking on headaches:

> *"Smoking raises carbon monoxide levels in the blood and brain, and carbon monoxide is known to cause headaches; smoking constricts blood vessels, contributing to headache and depriving brain tissues of essential oxygenation; and nicotine found in tobacco products is itself toxic to the brain and has an adverse effect on the liver."*

In addition, nicotine reduces the effectiveness of many headache medications and makes it more difficult to carry out healthful preventive practices such as exercise and relaxation. The Michigan Headache Institute recommends that all patients with frequent or recurrent headaches stop smoking as part of their treatment program and they strongly encourage a smoke-free environment at home and in the workplace.

Headache Triggers

Headache "triggers" may bring on a specific episode in someone who is prone to headaches. It is possible to eliminate many headache triggers by making lifestyle changes. It may take some effort, but the result may be far fewer or less severe headaches. Isn't it worth it? Below we'll discuss some common headache triggers.

DEHYDRATION

Dehydration is suspected to be a major cause of headaches. Our bodies are at least three-fourths water, and the brain is nearly 85% water; it detoxifies and cools itself by circulating body fluids. Therefore, when fluids are in short supply, both the body and the brain can easily become overwhelmed. A 2004 study showed that about 75% of Americans are suffering from chronic dehydration and that it can negatively affect health. Consuming large amounts of dehydrating beverages, including coffee, energy drinks, soda, and alcohol, in combination with consuming too little water, may lie at the heart of the problem. Is it really so difficult to drink enough water to keep our bodies healthy and help reduce the risk of headaches? Worldwide, access to clean, safe, drinkable water is a serious public health problem, but in developed countries, pure, filtered water comes right from the tap. Drink up! The question of how much to drink has been debated for decades. Here are some tips to help you meet your H2O requirements, *and* avoid headaches:

- We need to consume *at least* 1,500 mL of water every day just to replace body fluids lost through normal metabolic processes.
- We need to drink more water during warm weather, when we have a fever, when we exercise vigorously, and when we consume dehydrating foods and beverages.
- Older adults and seniors have a less pronounced thirst sensation and may need to be reminded to drink more water.
- One simple way to gauge ample water intake is to drink enough to maintain clear, light yellow urine. Dark-colored urine is far too

concentrated. It's hard on the kidneys and bladder, and it's a sign that you aren't drinking enough.

- People with special health considerations, such as kidney disease or heart conditions, should discuss appropriate fluid intake with their doctor.
- Electrolyte water, sports drinks, and coconut water help to keep electrolytes balanced when consuming extra fluids and are good choices for those who don't like plain water.
- Carry water with you as you travel and go about your work day. Keep a full glass on your desk that you can sip from throughout the day. Stop by the water fountain each time you use the bathroom.
- Drink before and after you exercise—including gardening and yard work outside in the sunshine. Teach toddlers from an early age to drink water to quench their thirst. They'll reap the benefits of fewer cavities and a decreased risk of childhood obesity because a popular alternative, juice, is high in sugar. Encourage schools to substitute bottled water for sugary sports drinks and soda, or send your child to school with a water bottle.
- Moderate your consumption of alcohol or give it up altogether. If you do drink alcohol on special occasions, be sure to drink plenty of water along with your alcoholic beverage.

SLEEP-ASSOCIATED FACTORS

Two studies have identified poor sleep as a risk factor in the development of chronic headaches. In one study, patients who reported the worst insomnia also suffered the highest risk for chronic headache when interviewed 11 years after initial assessment. A large Danish study found a correlation between short night-time sleep and tension-type headache. Studies have also looked at the association between habitual snoring which disrupts sleep as a risk factor for chronic daily headache. We don't yet know whether improving sleep patterns would necessarily decrease this risk, because that type of study has not yet been completed. It is an interesting area of research, which might ultimately lead to defining sleep requirements so that fewer numbers of people go on to develop chronic headaches. While we wait for research to catch up, anecdotal evidence certainly seems to indicate that changes in one's waking and sleeping routine can be an important and common headache trigger. Sleep is perhaps especially important in children (see Chapter 8), and helping or encouraging a child to fall asleep can often lead to a resolution of the headache. To summarize, maintaining a consistent sleep schedule, getting adequate restful sleep, and incorporating relaxation into bedtime routines may help to reduce headache frequency.

Another common sleep-related headache trigger is "jet lag." Coast-to-coast travel that crosses several time zones can throw our internal biological clocks out of sync, creating jet lag. The distance travelled is not as important as the direction, and the consensus seems to be that flying from west to east results in a greater tendency toward jet lag. Symptoms vary, but headache, fatigue, grogginess, irritability, and constipation are prominent.

HORMONES

Hormonal fluctuations, particularly in estrogens, seem to trigger headaches in many women, beginning in puberty and sometimes decreasing significantly during pregnancy and after menopause. Hormones may play other roles in the development and persistence of headaches in women, and I believe this area deserves more attention by the research

What Nurses Know...

Experienced flyers plan ahead and may even attempt to begin adapting to the destination time zone by going to sleep a little earlier, and waking a little earlier, for several days before flying. During flight, it is very important to avoid dehydration, which is why flight attendants encourage passengers to drink liquids frequently. On arrival, it's best to avoid caffeine and begin eating and sleeping at the accustomed local time. Walking outdoors, breathing fresh air, and enjoying as much sunlight as possible during the day will also help your body adapt.

community. The relationship between hormones and headaches in women including possible solutions are discussed in Chapter 9.

ENVIRONMENTAL HEADACHE TRIGGERS

Many headache sufferers will tell you that even fairly minor environmental changes, such as a drop in barometric pressure or a cold front coming in, can trigger a headache—and studies have shown this to be true for a relatively small number of headache sufferers. Temperature extremes and high humidity may be partially to blame. Similarly, exposure to carbon monoxide, cigarette smoke, and strong odors or perfumes is a well-known headache trigger. For many people, changing elevation (or altitude) is a powerful headache trigger. Altitude-induced headaches will often persist until the person descends to a lower elevation, and this is true for those frequenting mountain ski resorts as well those climbing Himalayan peaks.

But one important headache trigger we hear little about is a form of life that likes to grow in damp places with poor air circulation: mold. These members of the Fungi Kingdom release tiny, microscopic spores as part of their process of reproduction. If inhaled, these spores can be perceived by the immune system as foreign substances, resulting in an immediate or delayed hypersensitivity reaction and the release of histamine and other inflammatory substances. Histamine, in turn, may be responsible for producing such symptoms as sneezing, runny nose, and headache. Species of *Penicillum*, *Alternaria*, *Aspergillus*, *Cladosporium*, *Mucor*, and *Rhizopus* are among the environmental molds that can cause headaches, asthma, and other symptoms in sensitive people. Infants, young children, people with weakened immune systems, patients with chronic lung disease, and the elderly are at increased risk of mold-related health problems. Sinus and upper respiratory infections can be associated with mold exposure.

Some molds can cause breathing problems and toxic reactions that affect the nervous system. You may have heard of the dreaded "black mold" *Stachybotrys sp.*, which has caused severe illness in some families and made some homes uninhabitable. In some cases, black mold toxicity can be deadly if not treated promptly. So the question is, what can you do if this happens to your home or someone in your family?

It's possible to have an expert evaluate and treat your home for a mold problem using special mold remediation techniques. But this process is expensive and not always successful. A far better approach is to use prevention techniques. Be on the lookout for mold and take steps to eliminate it immediately. Make sure moisture isn't entering your home through a leaky roof or basement and fix all leaking pipes. If you live in a humid area, use a room dehumidifier in a main living area or in your sleeping area to keep indoor humidity well below 55%. Provide adequate ventilation and be diligent in making sure all bathrooms and cooking areas are properly vented to the outdoors, not into an interior living space or attic. Use an air purifier, preferably one with a HEPA air filter, to decrease airborne mold particles. Some newer HVAC (heating, ventilating, and air conditioning) systems include HEPA filtration.

One of the most likely times of exposure to dangerous molds is when rehabbing an older home. Wear a close-fitting dust mask while cleaning and dusting. But wear a respirator when pulling up old bathroom flooring or tiles, pulling up linoleum or vinyl in a laundry room or kitchen, pulling up old carpeting, or when tearing out old drywall. You need to advise any workers in your home to do so as well. When remodeling, replace old bathroom carpeting with a nonporous surface. Often there is a characteristic odor associated with mold in the home, so use your nose to be a mold detective. Small areas of mold can be cleaned and killed using a simple solution of 1 cup bleach in 1 gallon of water. Do not add any other household cleaners to this solution as dangerous fumes may result.

SENSORY TRIGGERS

Sensory stimuli such as bright lights, sun glaring off car windshields, strobe effects, loud movies, gunfire, strong odors, and even perfume can trigger migraine headaches. When possible, it is best to avoid excessive sensory stimulation. We'll review these in greater detail in Chapter 7.

MEDICATION USE AND OVERUSE

Medications such as oral contraceptives, including both oral formulations and skin patches, and vasodilating substances, such as nitroglycerine, can provoke strong headaches. There are also numerous studies that indicate that overuse of acute symptomatic headache medications can lead to rebound headaches. This subject is discussed in depth in Chapter 10. When medications such as Indocin (indomethacin) are prescribed for headache prevention, missing a dose can cause a headache. Even some vitamin supplements, such as niacin and vitamin A, may result in headache when taken in excess. Take all medications as directed by your physician and do not exceed recommended dosages.

Next, I'll discuss the importance of diet in helping to prevent headache symptoms. As you'll learn, a large number of potential headache triggers, including specific foods, food additives, and even eating habits, may contribute to the frequency and severity of headaches.

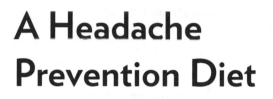

A Headache Prevention Diet

MSG triggers my headaches within 20 minutes, and some per-fumes trigger a headache within 20 seconds! I am a teacher of children who can't attend school, often for medical reasons, and I see often that problems in diet are contributing to their health problems. The suggestions I have made have improved the health of several children and their family members. One girl was having severe headaches and when I asked her whether she had eaten cheese within the past two days, she at first said no, and then remembered that she loves mac and cheese. When she stopped eating it, her headaches greatly diminished. Another student had been eating tons of beef jerky loaded with MSG. Even in the kids who don't seem to be listening to me I know I have planted the seed about diet. J.D.

Frequent headaches are often the result of triggers common to your daily routines. For many people, diet is an important and often overlooked headache trigger—as J.D.'s story illustrates—but it isn't just specific food triggers we need to consider. Headaches may also be related to poor diet, to skipping meals, or to fasting—which causes blood sugar to plummet. Many people have what is known as "functional hypoglycemia" and do best by eating smaller, regularly spaced meals and snacks throughout the day to help stabilize blood sugar levels. Unfortunately, many people who suffer from hypoglycemia remain undiagnosed. Dr. Alan Gaby, MD, has written that problems with blood sugar regulation "should be considered as a potential triggering factor in all migraine patients, particularly those who consume large amounts of refined carbohydrates or whose symptoms begin at a time of the day when blood glucose levels are typically lowest," which is usually late morning or late afternoon.

Food Allergies and Sensitivities that Contribute to Headaches

If you're sure you are eating regular, nutritious meals spaced throughout the day, then perhaps it is a good time to take a look at *what* you are eating and whether it could be affecting your headaches. One possible way in which diet influences headache development is through food allergy-induced inflammation. When our bodies are exposed to food proteins through our digestive system, these proteins are usually broken down into smaller fragments called peptides, and then broken down even further into individual amino acids. But when the body's immune system recognizes a certain food as harmful, or foreign, it can respond by creating antibodies to that food protein. Allergic reactions that occur very rapidly after eating an offending food involve the production of IgE antibodies. But new research on food allergies indicates that IgG antibodies, which are associated with a delayed, rather than immediate, reaction to foods we've consumed, may be to blame for inflammatory reactions that contribute to migraine headache.

The eight most common food allergens, which account for 90% of all food allergies, are peanuts, tree nuts, fish, shellfish, dairy products, soy, wheat, and eggs.

Corn and citrus fruits, like oranges, grapefruits, lemons and limes, are other common allergens. But our immune systems are capable of reacting to almost anything. Strawberries, sesame, chocolate, and even sugar can trigger allergic reactions. When we have an allergic reaction, the body releases inflammatory cytokines and some of these are capable of crossing the blood-brain barrier to contribute to headaches in sensitive individuals.

Recent studies have shown that childhood food allergies are twice as common as previously recognized. A survey of 38,000 children revealed that 8% suffered from at least one food allergy. Peanuts and peanut products affect children most often, followed by milk and shellfish. Tree nuts, eggs, fish, strawberries, wheat, and soy rounded out the top nine allergenic foods. Food allergies can range from mild to severe, or even deadly, and headache—including migraine—is a very common symptom. Food allergies are highest in preschool-age children, peaking at about age five, but teenage boys are also at risk for experiencing severe reactions.

But allergic reactions are not the only cause of food-induced headaches. Some specific foods contain vasoactive amines, substances that can constrict or dilate blood vessels the same way that certain medications can. Histamine is a vasoactive amine found in many common headache triggers, such as red wine and fermented foods.

Significance of Dietary Headache Triggers

Even though it's discussed frequently in the popular media, the subject of food sensitivities is very complex, and the ways in which foods and food additives affect those with headaches are even more difficult to understand. But for about 20% to 25% of headache sufferers, learning to identify food triggers can be life-changing. About one-quarter of migraine patients report that they are able to recognize food triggers. But according to Dr. Jeremy Kaslow, MD, who has written on the relationship between food sensitivities and headache,

> *"At the present time, food skin tests or RASTs [short for radioallergosorbent tests] are not sufficient predictors of which foods will cause headaches and are not indicated for screening patients with headaches. Skin and blood tests for allergies can be misleading since the headache is often not due to allergies but is a metabolic reaction. A food-headache diary is the most valuable*

way to determine which foods, if any, relate to your headaches. At least two weeks of complete avoidance is necessary before the relationship is clear."

Whether or not food sensitivities contribute significantly as headache triggers is a very controversial subject. Some neurologists have written of an "overemphasis" on dietary triggers of headaches, particularly migraine, while some alternative sources such as allergy expert Dr. James Braly and naturopathic physician and author Michael T. Murray cite dietary triggers as important triggers for headaches, particularly migraines. In researching this book, I have poured over dozens of books and hundreds of studies. I've spoken with many professionals and interviewed many patients. I have also drawn from my own experiences, and what I've learned is that there are many different headache triggers, and for some people these headache triggers can include: specific foods (wheat, gluten, eggs, and dairy products), food additives (MSG, sulfites), and certain substances found in some foods (like alcohol, tyramine, histamine, phenols, and phenylethalamine). This may be because some people do not produce sufficient enzymes to break down the amines these foods contain. People with migraines seem to be particularly vulnerable to amines. Learn more at this website: http://heartspring.net/migraine_headache_natural_treatments.html

These foods, food additives, and naturally occurring substances are not problematic for everyone who gets headaches, and, in fact, may not even be headache triggers all the time—even for someone who *is* sensitive to them during a headache cluster period, for example. The Michigan Headache Institute informational website makes the point that the potential for food triggers to provoke a headache is based on internal biological factors that determine an individual's vulnerability. Patients with migraine headaches seem to be especially vulnerable.

Let's look at some statistics. An older study published in the journal *Lancet* followed 60 patients with frequent migraines. These people were instructed to stop using oral contraceptives, tobacco, and the vasoconstricting drug ergotamine that is sometimes used for migraines, but they failed to improve. When these same people were placed on a strict food-elimination diet for 5 days, the results were impressive: Migraines disappeared within 5 days in a majority of patients. The elimination period was followed by the reintroduction of common foods while observing carefully for reactions. The foods to which patients reacted most strongly included the following: wheat (78% of patients), oranges (65% of patients), eggs (45% of patients), caffeinated beverages (40% of patients), chocolate and milk, (37% of patients reacted to each), beef (35% of patients), corn, cane sugar, and yeast (33% each), mushrooms (30% of patients), and peas (28% of patients).

Overall, the number of headaches in the study group decreased from over 400 per month to just 6 per month, and 85% of patients became headache-free. In a similar study involving 88 children, 93% recovered from migraine headaches following a restricted, low allergen diet. Again, a large number of patients reacted to specific foods. The most common reactions occurred with cow's milk (31% of patients), eggs (27%), oranges and wheat (24% reacted to each), and chocolate (25%). In addition, several food additives were found to provoke allergic reactions in children, including benzoic acid (a common food and beverage preservative) and tartrazine (a yellow food coloring). These studies are now nearly 30 years old and it would be interesting to repeat them, especially given the true increase in gluten intolerance and celiac disease. Headache is a well-documented, common symptom of wheat allergy, gluten sensitivity, and celiac disease.

Dr. Alan Gaby, MD, cites another piece of the food allergy and migraine puzzle: The drug Gastrocrom (cromolyn sodium), which is used to block allergies, was shown to prevent migraines in people who consumed foods known to provoke migraines. Despite these studies,

What Nurses Know...

There is no scientific evidence that everyone who gets headaches would benefit from eliminating specific problem foods. We are all unique and we must learn what our bodies are trying to tell us, often via the messenger headache.

there is still no agreement in the medical community on food allergy as a major cause of migraine or most other headache types. But like many of you, I know with absolute certainty that certain problem foods trigger my headaches and that staying away from these foods can greatly diminish the frequency of my headaches and eliminate the most severe headaches.

Specific Trigger Foods

The following are some triggers that are thought to cause headaches.

ALCOHOL USE

Alcohol is a common trigger for migraine and cluster headaches because it is a potent vasodilator, expanding blood vessels in as little as 45 minutes. Some alcoholic beverages contain high levels of the vasoactive amino acid tyramine and many people have complained of feeling a dull, hangover-type headache after drinking red wine, chardonnay (a white wine), or beer. Various other substances found in alcoholic beverages, including histamines and sulfites, may also contribute to an alcohol-induced headache. A 2008 study showed that even modest alcohol use may lead to decreased brain volume, perhaps because alcohol is "known to dehydrate tissues, and constant dehydration can have negative effects on any sensitive tissue," said the lead author Dr. Carol Ann Paul. The brain is particularly vulnerable to dehydration, and there is a clear relationship between dehydration and headaches.

ARTIFICIAL SUGARS (ASPARTAME AND SUCRALOSE)

Aspartame, also known as "Nutrasweet," is present in many artificially sweetened beverages and diet foods, including the sugar-substitute "Equal." In several studies, aspartame was associated with increased headache frequency and some in the epilepsy community fear it may increase the risk of seizure. Use of the sugar-substitute "sucralose" was associated with increased risk of migraine. Aspartame and sucralose contain no calories or nutrients and there are more healthful alternatives to consider, including naturally sweet fruit juices.

CAFFEINE

Caffeine is only one of many alkaloid substances found in coffee; black, green, and white teas; yerba mate herbal tea; cola soft drinks; and chocolate. It is also a common ingredient in energy drinks and both over-the-counter (OTC) and prescription medicines. Caffeine has a powerful influence on blood vessel constriction and is well known as both a headache trigger and, in some cases, as an acute headache treatment. Headaches can appear when you are drinking *too much* caffeine, or, if you are trying to *withdraw* from caffeine. It is also common for some patients to suffer from caffeine-withdrawal headaches when fasting prior to, during, and immediately after surgery, a fact I became well aware of when working as a postoperative nurse.

> *Nurse: Good morning, how are you feeling?*
> *Patient: Ugh ... COFFEE!!!*

Caffeine is one of the only known food substances that can, in fact, create a withdrawal headache—estimated to occur within 8 to 16 hours following consumption. Table 3.1 contains a list of the caffeine content of some common beverages, foods, and even medicines.

If you decide to remove caffeine from your diet, you must be aware of the very real withdrawal symptoms you are likely to experience, often including severe headache. Tapering off caffeine slowly is best. If you're a coffee drinker, an easy way to do this is to switch to "half-caff" by mixing decaffeinated and regular coffee, then gradually reducing the amount of regular coffee. Beverages to substitute for coffee or other caffeinated hot drinks include steamers made from milk or milk-alternatives, hot water with lemon and honey, and a variety of flavorful herbal teas.

CITRUS FRUITS

Oranges, tangerines, grapefruits, lemons, limes, and other related fruits can be headache triggers in certain individuals. Although allergy to citrus fruits is common, some people find they only have problems when they drink commercially produced orange juice. The reason for this may be that the rind can release the compound synephrine, which is a vasoconstrictor associated with migraine headache. Citrus fruits also contain histamine, to which headache sufferers may be particularly sensitive.

Table 3.1 Caffeine Content in Foods, Beverages, and Pharmaceuticals

Item	Serving Size	Caffeine (mg)
Starbucks grande coffee	16 oz.	330
Maximum Strength No-Doz	8 oz.	200
Dunkin' Donuts regular coffee	14 oz.	178
AMP Overdrive energy drink	16 oz.	160
Excedrin Extra Strength	2 tablets	130
Red Bull energy drink	12 oz.	114
Starbucks Tazo chai latte (grande)	16 oz.	100
Instant coffee	8 oz.	93
Ben & Jerry's Coffee Heath Bar Crunch	8 oz.	84
Rockstar Energy Drink	8 oz.	80
Jolt cola	12 oz.	72
Anacin Maximum Strength	2 tablets	64
Häagen-Dazs coffee ice cream	8 oz.	58
Mountain Dew soda	12 oz.	54
Brewed black tea (generic)	8 oz.	53
SoBe Essential Energy	8 oz.	48
Dr. Pepper soda	12 oz.	42
Snapple lemon iced tea	16 oz.	42
Pepsi	12 oz.	38
Yerba mate tea	8 oz.	38
Coke	12 oz.	35
Hershey's Special Dark chocolate bar	1.5 oz.	33
Arizona iced tea (black)	16 oz.	32
Nestea iced tea	12 oz.	26

DAIRY PRODUCTS

Foods made from cow's milk or from sheep's or goat's milk, including yogurt, buttermilk, whole and lower-fat content milks, ice cream, and cheese, trigger headaches in many people. Cow's milk is one of the top eight allergens. It is also mucous-producing and can cause sinus congestion which may lead to sinus headaches in sensitive individuals.

HISTAMINE

Alcohol can be a powerful headache trigger in itself, but red wine and beer are also high in inflammatory histamine, which can precipitate vascular headaches and migraine. Just recently, a new strain of yeast was developed at the University of British Columbia for use in the wine industry, aimed at reducing the amines in red wines and chardonnay that trigger headaches, spikes in blood pressure, and migraines. Food scientist Hennie van Vuuren, who spent 15 years on the project says, "about 30 per cent of the people in the world are sensitive to biogenic amines like histamines," and he includes himself in this group. Winemakers using the new yeast, labeled ML01, may not publicize it and are not required to disclose it on the label, fearing public backlash regarding concerns about genetic modification.

Fermented foods, chocolate, egg whites, strawberries, tomatoes, and citrus fruits also contain or release histamine that may induce headaches. Fish and shellfish tend to release significant amounts of histamine as they age. This is why you may be able to tolerate absolutely freshly caught or frozen seafood on one occasion, while on another occasion these same foods may trigger a headache. They can also increase heart rate, cause a runny nose, and produce a flushed face. When it comes to seafood, fresh is best.

MONOSODIUM GLUTAMATE

Monosodium glutamate (MSG), a flavor enhancer commonly used in some Asian foods, snack foods such as flavored chips and dry-roasted peanuts, frozen dinners, and seasoning salts can be a headache trigger. MSG may also be variously listed as hydrolyzed protein, glutamate, glutamic acid, or autolyzed yeast extract.

NITRITES

Processed meats like hot dogs, sausages, bologna, salami, and pastrami, cured and canned hams, smoked fish, and beef jerky often contain nitrites, yet another headache trigger.

PHENOLS/PHENOLIC COMPOUNDS

Phenolic compounds occur in a large number of plant foods. In growing plants, they help to protect cells from disease and the damaging effects of sunlight. Most foods high in phenols are also great antioxidants and they tend to include some of our healthiest, brightly colored fruits and vegetables like red cabbage, kale, tomatoes, and broccoli. Among fruits, berries tend to have the highest levels of phenols. But for some sensitive people, eating large amounts of foods that are very high in phenols, like yellow onions, soybeans, peanuts, coffee, green tea, and red wine can cause headaches.

PHENYLETHALAMINE

Phenylethalamine (PEA) is a vasoactive amine found in chocolate, some cheeses, and red wines. It is a rapidly metabolized, stimulating neurotransmitter. Ingesting alcohol, THC (found in marijuana), or a monoamine oxidase inhibitor (MAOI—a class of antidepressant) may lead to increased levels of phenylethalamine in the brain. Some people take a supplemental form of PEA to enhance mood, but in other people, PEA can provoke migraine-like headache symptoms. In animal studies, PEA produced significant changes in cerebral blood flow, mimicking the pattern of vascular changes that take place during a migraine attack.

SALT—SODIUM CHLORIDE

Eating high-salt foods in large quantities may lead to a migraine headache later in the day. One reason for this may be that too much salt can be dehydrating to the body and to the brain. In a 1979 study, migraine attacks were alleviated or reduced in a small number of patients who avoided salted snack foods for 6 months. It's easy enough to determine if excess salt is contributing to your headaches. Don't add extra salt to the foods you cook, and check all labels carefully for sodium content. You may be surprised by how much salt you and your family are actually consuming on a daily basis! Keep track of your diet, and your headaches, in a diary and see if reducing salt consumption makes a difference.

SUGAR

Especially in excess, cane sugar found in baked goods, candies, and desserts can trigger headaches. It may simply be "too much of a good thing," an allergy to cane sugar, or other sugar sensitivity. I often get headache after consuming sweets, especially on an empty stomach. But I can tolerate a small amount when consumed with protein-rich, healthier foods. A 1979 study published in the journal *Lancet* found cane sugar to be one of the most common triggers of migraine headache.

SULFITES

Naturally occurring sulfites found in onions, garlic, and other members of the allium family may trigger headaches in sensitive people. Sulfites are also commonly used to preserve foods such as dried fruits, potato products, food starches, snack foods, dough conditioner, cocktail shrimp, and jams and jellies.

Sulfites are used in a variety of ways, even as a fungicide to prevent gray mold on table grapes. One common source of sulfites is, again, red wine. Alternate names that indicate sulfite content include sulfur dioxide, sodium sulfite, sodium bisulfite, potassium bisulfate, sodium metabisulfate, and potassium sulfate.

TYRAMINE

Derived from the amino acid tyrosine, the compound tyramine is found both in the human body and in some common protein-rich and aged foods, including chocolate, mature cheeses like cheddar and Parmesan, sour cream, pickled herring, soy sauce, yogurt, overripe bananas, avocados, some yeast extracts, eggs, wheat, fava beans, and peanuts.

Tyramine is vasoactive, meaning that it has the capacity to influence the constriction of blood vessels, thus increasing blood pressure.

This effect can be especially dangerous if a person is taking an MAOI antidepressant, possibly resulting in a dangerous elevation in blood pressure. High dietary intake of tyramine may be linked with migraine headache. Several recent studies have found increased levels of circulating neurotransmitters in parts of the brain, including tyramine and related compounds, in both migraine and cluster headache.

WHEAT/GLUTEN

Grains like wheat, barley, rye, spelt, kamut, and faro contain a difficult-to-digest protein complex referred to as "gluten." For some people who are gluten intolerant, including those who have celiac disease, eating foods made from gluten-containing grains can be a powerful headache trigger. Others react to the yeast used in many raised baked goods. We'll focus more specifically on the relationship between celiac disease and increased frequency of migraine, in particular, in the section below.

Celiac Disease and Headaches

Celiac disease is an important, often overlooked, cause for frequent headaches, especially in children. Celiac disease is a genetic autoimmune disorder triggered by consuming certain proteins found in wheat, barley, rye, and related grains—collectively known as "gluten." Celiac disease causes inflammation and flattening of the intestinal villi—the carpet-like absorptive surface of the small intestine—leading to nutrient deficiencies and multiple health effects throughout

What Nurses Know...

An easy way to remember five common categories of foods thought to be associated with headaches, and migraines in particular, is to think of the letter "C": cheese, chocolate, coffee, cola, and citrus.

the body (not just diarrhea and failure to thrive as once thought). Episodic headaches, sometimes accompanied by temporary neurological effects, may be triggered by the immune system's inflammatory reaction to consuming gluten. A 2009 study published in the *Journal of Pediatric Gastroenterology & Nutrition* looked at the prevalence of undiagnosed celiac disease in a large number of children with headaches. They also surveyed children recently diagnosed with celiac disease for symptoms of headache before and after beginning a gluten-free diet, the recommended treatment for celiac disease. Of the children with celiac disease, 77.3% reported significant improvement in their headaches, and 27.3% were completely headache-free after beginning the gluten-free diet. In the group of children with headaches, screening for celiac disease led to a positive diagnosis in 5%, which is about five times the rate in the U.S. population. Having worked with many children with celiac disease who present with an astonishing array of symptoms often including headaches, I believe that screening children with frequent headaches for this disorder is very important. Although Toni, who tells her story below, did not discover that she had celiac disease as a child, she began experiencing symptoms many years before she was diagnosed.

From the age of 12 I had chronic constipation, sensitive skin, and a pasty complexion. I had my first migraine at age 19—it began with a loss of peripheral vision for approximately two hours, followed by a bad headache and nausea. This occurred three more

What Nurses Know...

People with frequent or chronic headaches, or other symptoms of celiac disease, should know that even if past blood tests have been negative, it does not hurt to repeat testing, because techniques and accuracy have improved markedly in the past decade. For more information on celiac disease please see the University of Maryland Center for Celiac Research's public website: www. celiaccenter.org times in a one-year period. At approximately age 27, I developed severe stomach cramping that would begin late in the day on most days of the week. It never seemed clear what was causing this and it was determined to be stress-related by a family physician. Meanwhile, the migraines were still occurring up to several times per year. At around age 30 I began having a "basic headache" [not a migraine] anywhere from 3 to 6 days per week. In addition, my gastrointestinal symptoms were increasing, although masked by the use of antacids, antigas medications, and avoiding large meals.

Finally, at the age of 31, I was diagnosed with celiac disease and began to eat, and continue to eat, 100% gluten-free. I now only experience a migraine about once a year and have identified current triggers to be neck and upper back tension. I have found that my neck, shoulder, and muscles throughout my scalp are very sensitive to increased strain. I still tend to get at least one "basic headache" per week that doesn't last very long and can be alleviated with ibuprofen.

—TONI

It isn't possible to eliminate all of the foods that might possibly trigger a headache and still eat a healthy, well-balanced diet. Diets that are too restrictive are also too difficult for most people to follow and they can even result in nutritional deficiencies if followed for an extended period of time. Keeping a diet diary is key to helping you identify your individual food triggers and plan a healthy diet that also may reduce your headache frequency.

Essential Elements of a Headache-Prevention Diet

Can diet also be used *positively* to help prevent headaches? The answer is probably "Yes." However, as you can see from the large number of possible headache-trigger foods, a one-size-fits-all headache-prevention diet will simply not work. We each need to discover our individual food sensitivities (or food allergies) and avoid those foods. Probably the best plan is to begin with a "food elimination diet" by excluding all but a small number of foods which are the least likely to cause a reaction, and gradually re-introducing other foods one by one. Such a diet will yield useful results only if you follow it strictly and avoid introducing more than one food every three days— so, it takes patience. And remember, strict food elimination diets should not be followed when pregnant or nursing, or at the expense of general health.

More generally, eating foods high in magnesium, like fresh fish, beans, bran flakes, and dark, leafy greens, or adding a magnesium supplement may help to reduce headache frequency, especially if you are prone to migraines. Eating more foods high in antiinflammatory Omega-3 fatty acids, such as cold water ocean fish like salmon, tuna, sardines, herring, mackerel, and halibut may help to reduce headache severity (see Chapter 5). Omega-3 fatty acids are also available from fish oil, krill oil, and flax-seed oil. Another plant-based antiinflammatory is gamma-linoleic acid, found in evening primrose, black current, and borage oils. Be sure to discuss any dietary changes, including the use of dietary supplements, with your doctor first.

Next, we'll discuss how to find appropriate care for your headaches, and building your health care team. As you'll learn, there are plenty of options for finding professional help, and relief.

What Nurses Know...

Fish oil has anticoagulant effects and should not be used if you have a bleeding disorder or are planning to have surgery.

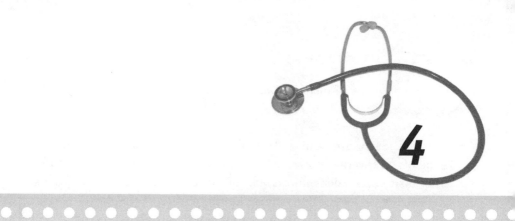

Finding Help for Your Headaches

I went to my general practitioner, a chronic pain specialist, an osteopath, and a headache specialist before I finally found the right person to treat my headaches. This new doctor, also a headache specialist, was sympathetic—perhaps because she also suffers from migraines. We were about the same age so I knew she was familiar with some of the factors in my headaches, like fluctuating hormone levels. She immediately agreed that I needed an effective rescue medication, but she did not stop there. My doctor ordered imaging to rule out any serious indicators. She shared with me that she sees headache management as a challenge, that she is persistent, and that she is willing to explore many possibilities in an effort to obtain pain relief and reduce headache frequency. Over time, I've come to appreciate that my doctor understands that headache patterns can change, which means management strategies must also change. She stays on top of her research and continues to love her job as a neurologist. And I benefit from her enthusiasm and expertise by receiving the best possible care.   JOANNA

Many headache specialists stress that successful headache treatment depends on several factors, most importantly, the physician's accurate diagnosis—which depends on *your* accurate description of symptoms. An equally important factor may be the nature of the doctor-patient relationship, which must be open and honest, with trust on the part of both patient and physician. Your physician must trust that you are telling the truth about your symptoms, and believe you. In turn, you must tell the truth without exaggeration or hyperbole. You must also use your medications as prescribed, or admit that you did not. Otherwise, it will be impossible for your physician to be certain whether a particular treatment plan is, or is not, successful. It may help to remember that diagnosing and managing headache pain is one of the most demanding challenges in neurology, made more so by its often chronic nature and the sheer numbers of people who get headaches.

The Challenge of Diagnosing Headaches

The first step in being a good headache patient is to be a good historian, and one of the best tools to ensure accuracy in reporting your symptoms and your response to treatment is to keep a headache diary. Your doctor will use this information to both evaluate the symptoms of an individual headache attack and to look for patterns in your headaches over time. I have included a sample headache diary in the

What Nurses Know...

THERE'S AN APP FOR THAT!

Keeping your headache diary on a simple computer spreadsheet is an easy method, and there are now even headache diary applications such as iHeadache for the iPhone, iPod Touch, and Blackberry.

Appendix. You can use this to make copies or follow its example in creating your own.

Even with your best efforts to provide your physician with an accurate record of your symptoms and your response to medications and other treatment, obtaining an accurate diagnosis can sometimes be difficult. Writer Paula Kamen, a chronic headache patient and author, shares her personal story in her book *All in My Head.* In the course of her 15 years or so of dealing with chronic pain, she has been diagnosed with atypical migraine, tension headache, mixed headache (combination migraine and tension headache), chronic daily headache, and chronic tension-type headache. How can this happen? Well, it's complicated. Let's look at some of the things that might influence your diagnosis.

First, headaches are invisible, with hidden symptoms that you can feel subjectively, but very few objective signs for your physician to use in diagnosis. In migraines the vast majority of MRI or other imaging scans show no evidence of an organic brain abnormality. Second, over time, your symptoms might add up to better fit an alternate diagnosis. Your response to certain medications may help to narrow the diagnosis. Or, experts in the headache field may create an entirely new headache category, as happened to writer Paula Kamen with the new classification of "chronic daily headache." There may also be instances where different physicians that you see offer different diagnoses. Stay calm and try to have an open discussion with each physician, focusing on the treatment plans suggested and the reasons given for prescribed medications or other, nonmedical treatments. Ask about the risks and benefits of each, as well as about alternatives. When in doubt, you can always seek another opinion, perhaps from a physician with a different expertise—such as a chronic pain specialist.

A Comprehensive Physical Examination: What to Expect

Any doctor who sees you for complaint of a persistent, severe, or chronic headache should do a complete neurological examination to help rule out most abnormalities associated with secondary headaches caused by a disease. It is a time-honored process and doesn't take long unless there are signs of a possible problem that needs ferreting out.

A thorough physical exam should evaluate your cardiovascular status as well, including heart rate, heart rhythm, and blood pressure. This may also involve listening for abnormalities in the blood flow through your carotid arteries. A musculoskeletal exam should assess your range of motion, particularly in the upper spine and neck, your temporomandibular joints (TMJ), and the various groups of associated muscles on either side of your neck, throat, back of the head, jaw, and forehead. Your doctor may ask you to flex your neck to assess for stiffness or pain. Assessing your motor reflexes and gait may help to rule out other neurological illnesses. Briefly shining a bright light in your eyes, asking you to look up, down, and to the side; to blink; and to follow a moving object helps to assess the function of the cranial and optic nerves. Your doctor will also ask you to describe any visual abnormalities, such as visual field cuts, dark spots, or floaters. I hope you will use this expectation to do your own screening, determining whether the doctor you are seeing for the first time is as thorough as you would like. If you are suffering from a severe, debilitating, chronic headache pain, a thorough neurological and physical exam is important, and as a patient it is precisely what you need and deserve.

Neuroimaging: Diagnostic Imaging for Headaches

An MRI or CT of the head and brain is not required to diagnose most primary headaches but may be ordered for unusual headaches or when a more serious cause is suspected for secondary headaches. For example, imaging can help to rule out life-threatening brain tumors and strokes—both of which include headache symptoms. It bears repetition here that your headache history is the most important factor in both diagnosis and treatment. Your doctor will examine your headache history or diary, and in combination with a physical exam, determine whether there is an identifiable cause for your headaches. Physicians must rule out structural abnormalities of the head, jaw, and neck; metabolic disorders that may be contributing to your headaches; and consider problems related to your past medical history such as traumatic head injury. After that, the doctor uses his or her own judgment to decide whether neuroimaging is necessary. You may need preauthorization from your insurance company for this. The American Academy of Neurology (AAN)

Physician Guidelines suggesting the need for neuroimaging in headache patients include:

- A new daily headache or near-daily headache that does not quite fit the diagnosis criteria for a primary headache disorder
- Family history or medical history that increases the risk of disease-based neurological cause of a secondary headache
- An abnormal neurological exam combined with patient's headache history
- Unusual symptoms of a new headache or worrisome changes in previous headache pattern that raise suspicion, such as: headaches that awaken patients from sleep, headaches following head trauma, headaches consistently triggered by exertion, headaches in patients with abnormal heart rate and blood pressure, and new headaches in young children under age five or older patients over age fifty

In summary, not all headaches require diagnostic imaging. However, neuroimaging is a valuable tool in diagnosing the rarer types of headache and new onset cough-induced and exertional headaches. The most common types of diagnostic imaging for headaches are discussed below.

CT/CAT SCAN

Computed tomography, or the CT scan, is a noninvasive test that may help your neurologist or headache specialist locate, or rule out, serious causes of head and facial pain such as a sinus abscess, an infection in the brain, or swelling. CT scans are also preferred to MRI for diagnosing bleeding in the brain. CT scans use a large, revolving x-ray ring that rotates around the head, making a high-speed "whirring" sound. As the x-ray beams rotate around the circumference of the head, sensitive detectors gather and relay information to a computer which converts it into visual slices, or cross-sections. CT scans are able to provide details about organs, soft tissues, and blood vessels, and are able to provide a consistently readable *three-dimensional* picture of the brain. Normal x-rays show only two-dimensional images with overlapping structures. From a patient's perspective the CT scan is less confining than the MRI "tube." A CT is sometimes performed with a contrast medium given intravenously (IV) to provide a more detailed image.

Before scheduling the exam, be sure that your doctor is aware of all the medications you are taking, especially beta-blockers or the diabetes drug Glucophage (metformin), and that he or she knows about any recent illnesses or chronic medical conditions including heart disease, asthma, diabetes, kidney disease, or thyroid problems, as these can increase the risk of adverse effects. Women should always inform both their doctor and the exam technician if there is even a remote possibility that they could be pregnant. Always let both your doctor and the radiology technician know if you have any allergies, especially, of course, to the contrast dye. Patients may have been told in the past that an allergy to shellfish or iodine increases the likelihood of an allergic reaction to IV contrast, but multiple reliable sources say this simply isn't true. People with seafood allergies are reacting to proteins in the item being consumed, and IV contrast material does not contain any allergic antibodies. Similarly, iodine sensitivity appears to carry little risk.

However, reactions to radioactive contrast material (RCM) are fairly common, occurring in 5% to 8% of patients. This is due to RCM's direct action on the body's mast cells, which can release histamine and other inflammatory chemicals. A mild reaction includes experiencing an uncomfortable feeling of warmth, nausea, and vomiting which lasts a short time and does not require treatment. Stronger reactions, including protracted vomiting and hives, occur in less than 1% of patients. Life-threatening anaphylaxis is very rare, affecting 0.1% of patients receiving RCM. The elderly appear to have a higher risk of severe reactions to IV contrast materials.

Diagnostic imaging is conducted in a medical facility and should a reaction occur it will be treated immediately and appropriately with injected epinephrine and strong antihistamines, as well as the use of IV fluids as necessary. This lessens any risk to patients considerably.

Patients can prepare for a CT by leaving all metal jewelry, hairpins, and barrettes at home and by wearing loose clothing. Removable bridges and other dental work should also be left at home. These are expensive items and you do not want to risk losing or damaging them. You may be asked to change into a gown, but for a head-CT, sometimes this isn't necessary. When you get to the exam area you will also have to leave behind your eye-glasses and sometimes even your hearing-aides. You may be asked to avoid eating or drinking anything for several hours prior to the CT, especially if contrast is being used. A CT of the head and brain usually takes about 30 to 40 minutes. After, or sometimes during, your exam, the images are reviewed and interpreted by a radiologist—a medical doctor who has had years of special training in interpreting these images.

MRI

MRI, or magnetic resonance imaging, uses pulses of radio waves and a controlled magnetic field instead of x-rays so no radiation is involved. This is one way in which MRI differs from CT. The brain selectively absorbs radio waves during many rapid pulses, emitting detectable radio signals that are collected, analyzed, and converted into detailed images by a powerful computer. MRI provides an even greater degree of resolution of the brain. Beyond removing all metal jewelry, there is no special preparation for MRI of the brain; you may eat and take medications prior to the exam.

You will be assisted to lie comfortably on a moveable platform, which will then slide into a confining tube or tunnel that emits the radio waves. This part can be a little claustrophobic, especially for patients with preexisting anxiety, but you need to lie perfectly still during the exam. There are several things that help patients to cope. First, it's important to know that at all times the technician administering the test will be able to see and hear you, and you will be able to hear them. They will check in with you every few minutes to let you know what to expect and to let you know how you are doing. For example, they may say, "Now you are going to hear a series of loud beeps. Please lie as still as you can and I'll let you know when we're done." Second, you may be offered ear plugs and/or close-fitting headphones that will play music of your choice. This usually helps to distract patients and reduce anxiety. It also helps to close your eyes and try to relax throughout the exam, which usually lasts about 20 to 45 minutes.

From a patient's perspective, undergoing an MRI of the brain has several distinct challenges, especially if you already have a headache. The most uncomfortable part of experiencing an MRI while you are experiencing a headache is the noise factor. Throughout the test, you will hear a rapping sound at different intervals and decibels, from a soft, rapid buzzing sound, to a series of loud knocks. For people with a severe headache this can, at times, sound and feel like a jackhammer in one's head, but the loudest portion of the test lasts a very short time. Follow your doctor's recommendation regarding taking prophylactic medication. For patients with high anxiety levels, a sedative or antianxiety medication is occasionally ordered to be given prior to MRI. If this is your expectation, you will need to arrange to have someone drive you home after your exam. Some specialized radiology centers have "open MRI" machines that have a much broader, shorter tunnel, and this helps greatly to reduce the sensation of claustrophobia in anxious patients.

THE PET SCAN

The PET scan, or positron emission tomography, is an expensive test that probably provides little value in the diagnosis of migraine or other primary headaches. But its three-dimensional color image showing brain *activity*, rather than structure, is sometimes used for research on migraine—especially in examining blood flow, measuring brain function, and viewing activity in specific areas of the brainstem. The test involves injecting a tiny amount of fluorine-based radio isotope which is absorbed by active brain tissues.

PET scans can also be used to detect some brain tumors and occasionally to check for tumor recurrence. A study in *The Southern Medical Journal* found PET scan to be useful in diagnosing giant cell arteritis (GCA), an inflammation of blood vessels affecting the temporal artery which can cause severe headache, scalp and facial tenderness, visual disturbances, and or wide spread muscle and body aches (learn more in Chapter 15).

Finding a Physician

What kind of doctor should you see? Unless you are in an emergency situation and need help right away, your family doctor or primary care physician is the best person to see about your headaches. Your doctor will make an initial assessment and perhaps offer adequate treatment for infrequent, tension-type headaches and migraine. After doing an exam, viewing your headache diary to look for patterns and frequency, and evaluating your response to treatment, your doctor may refer you to a neurologist, or to a headache specialist—a neurologist who deals exclusively with headaches. But you can also be your own advocate, and if the severity of your headaches is interfering substantially with your life, you can ask for a referral to a specialist, or depending on your insurance plan, seek out a board-certified specialist in neurology on your own.

For women with headaches that correspond with the menstrual cycle, it certainly wouldn't hurt to get some advice from a gynecologist. Hormonally-related headaches are often treated by gynecologists. You may also be experiencing side-effects related to a medication, like birth control pills or patches, which were prescribed by your gynecologist. Having this conversation might lead to a simple change in your treatment plan and a resolution of your headaches. Other specialists that might be involved in headache care include dentists for TMJ problems, and ear, nose, and throat specialists (ENTs) for sinus-related problems.

Headache Specialists and Specialty Clinics

One alternative for patients with severe or persistent headaches is to go straight to the top by visiting one of a small number of headache specialty clinics.

What Nurses Know...

Headache specialists are swamped, and you may have better luck getting a timely appointment if your doctor's office makes the call for you, which is a common practice. Even that is no guarantee and it may take months to get in to see a specialist, so planning ahead is essential. Of course, if you have warning signs of a serious or life-threatening health disorder, exceptions will be made because you need prompt or immediate care.

Table 4.1 Specialty Headache Clinics

| | Recommended Clinics and Medical Facilities | | | |
Facility	Location	Website	Adults	Children
Diamond Headache Clinic	Chicago, IL	www.diamondheadache.com	Yes	
Arkansas Children's Hospital—Headache Clinic	Little Rock, AR	www.archildrens.org		Yes
Brigham and Women's—Faulkner Hospital Headache Center	Boston, MA	www.brighamandwomens.org	Yes	
California Pacific Medical Center—Pediatric Headache Clinic	San Francisco, CA	http://cpmc.org/advanced/pediatrics/services		Yes
Carolina Headache Institute	Chapel Hill, NC	www.carolinaheadacheinstitute.com	Yes	
Children's Hospital Central California—The Neurology Practice	Madera, CA	www.childrenscentralcal.org/Services/medical/neurology		Yes
Children's National Medical Center—Headache Clinic	Washington, DC	www.childrensnational.org/DepartmentsandPrograms		Yes
Dent Neurological Institute	Amherst, NY	www.dentinstitute.com	Yes	
East Tennessee Children's Hospital	Knoxville, TN	www.etch.com		Yes
Headache Care Center	Springfield, MO	www.headachecare.com	Yes	
Headache Center at Cleveland Clinic	Cleveland, OH	http://my.clevelandclinic.org/headache_center	Yes	
Headache Center, Cincinnati Children's Hospital	Cincinnati, OH	www.cincinnatichildrens.org		Yes
Houston Headache Clinic	Houston, TX	http://houstonheadacheclinic.com	Yes	

Name	Location	Website		
Integrative Pain Center of Arizona	Tucson, AZ	www.ipcaz.org	Yes	
Jefferson Headache Center T.J. University Hospital	Philadelphia	www.jefferson.edu/headache	Yes	
Keeler Center for the Study of Headache	Ojai, CA	www.migrainecenter.org	Yes	
Mayo Clinic Rochester Minnesota	Rochester, MN	www.mayoclinic.org/neurology-rst/headachegroup	Yes	
Mayo Clinic Scottsdale Arizona	Scottsdale, AZ	www.mayoclinic.org/neurology-sct/	Yes	
Michigan Headache and Neurological Institute	Ann Arbor, MI	www.mhni.com	Yes	
Michigan Headache Clinic	East Lansing, MI	http://michiganheadache.com	Yes	
New England Center for the Headache	Stamford, CT	www.headachenech.com	Yes	
Phoenix Children's Hospital Headache Clinic	Phoenix, AZ	www.phoenixchildrens.com/medical specialties		Yes
Princeton and Rutgers Neurology	Princeton, NJ	www.princetonandrutgersneurology.com/services	Yes	
San Francisco Headache Clinic	San Francisco, CA	www.sfcrc.com/html/headache.htm	Yes	
St. Louis Children's Hospital Comprehensive Headache Center	St. Louis, MO	www.stlouischildren		Yes
Swedish Headache Center	Seattle, WA	www.swedish.org/body.cfm?id=1348	Yes	
The Children's Hospital (Denver Area)—Headache Clinic	Aurora, CO	www.thechildrenshospital.org		Yes

(Continued)

Table 4.1 Specialty Headache Clinics (Continued)

| | Recommended Clinics and Medical Facilities | | | |
Facility	Location	Website	Adults	Children
The Headache Center of Southern California	Oceanside, CA	http://the-headachecenter.com	Yes	
The Headache Center of Southern California	Oceanside, CA	www.the-headachecenter.com	Yes	
The Headache Institute at Roosevelt Hospital Center	New York, NY	www.wehealny.org/headache	Yes	
UCSF Headache Center at Divisadero	San Francisco, CA	www.ucsfhealth.org	Yes	
University Neurologists, PSC	Louisville, KY	www.faulknerhospital.org/programs_heacen.html	Yes	
University of California Davis Center for Pain Medicine	Sacramento, CA	www.ucdmc.ucdavis.edu/pain/	Yes	
University of California San Diego Center for Pain Medicine	La Jolla, CA	anes-cppm.ucsd.edu	Yes	
University of Chicago Medical Center Migraine Headache Clinic	Chicago, IL	www.uchospitals.edu/specialties/neurology/migraine	Yes	
University of Maryland Medical Center Pediatric Headache Clinic	Baltimore, MD	www.umm.edu/pediatrics		Yes
University of South Florida Headache and Pain Program	Tampa, FL	http://health.usf.edu/medicine/neurology	Yes	
University of Vermont Headache Clinic	Burlington, VT	www.med.uvm.edu/neurology	Yes	

Note: This is a wide-ranging, but not necessarily comprehensive, list. There may be a specialty clinic in your state.

Why a Holistic Approach is Necessary

Conventional medicine is an excellent choice for diagnosis, but when it comes to treatment, patients have some broader options. We've learned previously how stress, diet, and musculoskeletal factors play a role in headache development, so taking a holistic approach to treatment makes good sense. First, I would advise any chronic headache sufferer to take a look at their overall health. An examination of the rest of your body can yield useful information. As health practitioners in our fast-paced practices, we sometimes don't have enough time to look and listen to the extent we'd like to, and it is possible to miss things. We also don't have enough time for as much patient education as we think is ideal. Conventional medicine is expert in diagnosing and treating acute and emergency conditions, but possibly less expert in treating chronic illness, in which factors such as diet, stress, and lifestyle must be considered. However, things are improving rapidly and we are definitely moving in the right direction, especially with regard to the impact of stress, obesity, and sedentary lifestyle on health—areas which have received a lot of attention in recent years.

As headache sufferers, we're all individuals with our own bio-chemistry, and we're uniquely influenced by genetic factors and our

What Nurses Know...

TRAVELLING WITH CHRONIC HEADACHES

Take enough medication along for the trip, each in its original container. Also take along your physician's phone number in case of an emergency. Carrying a card with emergency contacts and medical information is always a good safety strategy. Remember that carrying large amounts of narcotic painkillers or benzodiazepine tranquilizers may be a problem in today's heightened security, so it may be helpful to carry a note from your physician and a contact number, especially if transporting these items.

environment as well. But there are some general principles that head-ache sufferers should consider in a comprehensive search for answers to chronic headache pain as well as whole-body wellness.

Seeing the Bigger Picture

Step away from your focus on headaches for a moment. What about the rest of you? Perhaps there are clues that you've been missing. Each of the areas discussed below may have some relationship to your headaches. And it's possible that several factors are working together to create the inflammation and pain in your body that you experi-ence as sporadic, frequent, or severe headaches. Consider all of the following:

1. *Breathing*: Starting with an essential activity, examine your breathing. Do you breathe deeply and fully, down into your abdo-men and pelvis, or are your inhalations confined to the chest? You may benefit from taking a yoga class. Yoga focuses on inte-grating breathing, stretching, and more athletic poses. You may also want to spend some time working with a breath therapist to learn diaphragmatic breathing. Learning to breathe properly can do wonders in controlling your stress level. Deep, relaxed, breath-ing calms the overstimulated sympathetic nervous system—which raises our heart rate and anxiety level—and helps to create a better balance with the parasympathetic nervous system. Our bodies do this naturally when we take a deep breath and let it out slowly, and yawn, stretch, or sigh. Activation of the parasympathetic nervous system is very good for health and healing.

2. *Appearance*: Take a good look in the mirror at your face, hair, and the skin over your entire body. Are there rashes, blemishes, dry skin, areas of hair loss or thinning hair, dark circles or bags under your eyes? These could be signs of chronic illness affecting your body or signs that your body is reacting to something in your envi-ronment. There are many systemic health problems that can be associated with headaches, including autoimmune disorders.

3. *Sleep*: Think about your ability to sleep restfully, for sleep is when our bodies heal, our nervous systems jettison the accumulated stresses of daily life, and our adrenals, part of our fight-or-flight

system, can recover. Are you able to fall asleep easily, sleep for at least 7-9 hours (in adults—or 8.5-11 hours in older children and teens) and wake feeling rested?

4. *Digestion*: Think about your digestion, your daily food intake, food preferences, food dislikes, and how you feel during periods *between* meals (light-headed, anxious?), and *after* meals (bloated, gassy, or drowsy?). Do you have any personal or family history of food allergy, food sensitivity, or celiac disease? This is another area to explore.

5. *Elimination*: Do you empty your bowels regularly? Do you have to run to the bathroom unexpectedly, or do you have to try every trick in the book to go at all? Do you know that constipation is reported by many patients to be a factor in triggering headaches?

6. *Energy Level*: What is your basic energy level? Are you able to accomplish all the things you want and need to do on a weekly basis? Are there days when you just need to lie in bed to recover? This may be a sign that you are suffering from chronic fatigue syndrome (CFS), hypothyroidism, anemia, or another health condition that may be influencing your headaches.

As you can see, this is a lot for any one doctor to take on—let alone have the time to help you put together a comprehensive treatment plan. This is why it may be a better option to use the knowledge obtained from your whole-body head-to-toe self-assessment to build a health care team of trusted professionals, each with knowledge from their particular field of expertise. It is helpful to have a primary care physician, a neurologist or headache specialist, and sometimes a naturopathic physician, physical therapist, or massage therapist, depending on your particular headache disorder. Alternative therapies might also be helpful, so I've included a comprehensive explanation of some of the therapies most useful in treating headaches in the next chapter.

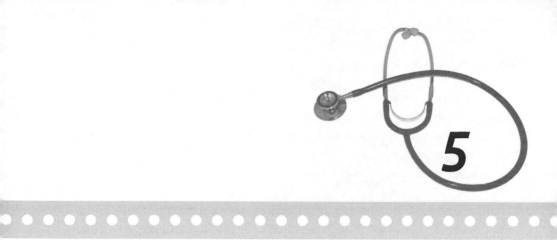

A Review of Alternative and Complementary Therapies

About five years ago I began experiencing frequent muscle tight-
ness and pain in my upper back, neck, and upper trapezius mus-
cle (the muscle just above the collar bone that connects the head
and shoulder). The discomfort would become worse throughout
the day, progressing to a one-sided migraine at the back of my
head, daily. Over a few months the pain became chronic, and I
developed occipital neuralgia—heightened nerve sensitivity and
an inability to tolerate the slightest pressure on the back of my
neck and head. Despite seeing conventional medicine doctors, my
pain became incapacitating and prevented me from living a nor-
mal life. The first time that I experienced significant relief was
following a session of craniosacral therapy, after which I was
completely headache-free for four or five days. This gave me hope
and prompted me further on my search, and I eventually had

gentle cervical manipulation using the NUCCA technique, followed by regular sessions of Integrative Manual Therapy (IMT) practiced by a very skilled physical therapist. Today I have been able to resume my life after missing out on so many things for nearly two years. WENDY

Conventional medicine is practiced by those with an MD (Medical Doctor) or DO (Doctor of Osteopathy) degree in medicine. Any practice that falls outside of these well-defined programs of medical education generally falls into the category of alternative medicine, which itself has many possible therapies to pursue. Well-accepted alternative medical practices are sometimes referred to as "complementary medicine," or variously, "Complementary and Alternative Medicine," or CAM. There is now a National Center for CAM Medicine (NCCAM), part of the National Institute of Health (NIH), which funds and publishes serious clinical research on the efficacy of nontraditional medicine.

CAM and an Integrative Approach

The past four decades or so have seen a gradual influx of alternative practitioners into the health care field. Some of these practices are relatively new, without much of a track record of proven success, and perhaps should be taken with a grain of salt. Others are ancient, with a record of practice going back thousands of years, but are relatively new to our Western culture. Acupuncture is a popular example, one that has grown to be accepted by the medical community, and even health care insurers, for its efficacy in treating many health disorders—but perhaps especially, pain.

One commonality among these complementary therapies is that they often take a broader, holistic approach to health, taking in physical, psychological, spiritual, and environmental information both in diagnosis and in developing a treatment plan. Since its earliest beginnings, nursing has held this view. Nursing care plans address the total care of the patient, and often the patient's family as well, including psychological and social needs.

In a recent review of CAM therapies in the well-respected journal *Headache*, the authors concluded, "There is a growing role for CAM

What Nurses Know...

When conventional and CAM approaches are used together, it is referred to as "integrative medicine"—a highly practical newer practice that allows patients to see a variety of doctors and other health care practitioners in the same office. More and more, practitioners are learning to work together to give their patients the best in acute health care, preventive medicine, and wellness.

treatment in the multidisciplinary management of headache disorders. In addition to their potential in decreasing headache frequency and intensity, these modalities also serve to provide the patient with a greater sense of self-efficacy."

I'll review some of the most promising or useful CAM therapies offering relief for headaches and their associated symptoms. One drawback is that some of these therapies are not commonly covered by insurance, and patients must pay out-of-pocket, frequently at the time of service. Others are covered if ordered by an MD or DO for a specified treatment interval. But you will need to check with your insurer to see what services are covered, as plans and coverage vary.

ACUPUNCTURE

Acupuncture is hugely popular and there are now more than 10,000 licensed acupuncturists in the United States. I personally have experienced complete and near-instantaneous migraine relief from a single properly placed acupuncture needle, and I know many people who are strong advocates of this ancient practice. So much research has been published regarding acupuncture's effectiveness on a variety of headaches that it was almost impossible to condense it into a few paragraphs. But the research on acupuncture and headaches is actually very promising.

Acupuncture was developed in China thousands of years ago. This practice uses disposable, thin, sterile-needles that are inserted

into the body at specific "acupoints" located along 14 energetic acupuncture channels, or "meridians," corresponding somewhat to
the body's major organs. Although it is superficially invasive, it is
not usually painful—most patients find the therapy to be relaxing.
More than 2 million people in the United States are estimated to be
receiving regular acupuncture and about 10% of them are headache
patients.

In traditional Chinese medicine, headaches follow one of nine possible patterns, including the "wind cold pattern," in which a headache
accompanies an upper respiratory virus, and the "Qi (vital energy)
stagnation pattern," associated with premenstrual headaches accompanied by mood swings and breast tenderness. Migraine headaches
are associated with a "liver yang rising pattern," frequently related to
stress, and key symptoms can include anxiety, insomnia, and visual
disturbances. The upper cervical acupoints are frequently used to
treat headaches, and there are specific healing herbs associated with
each headache pattern.

Acupuncture has been successfully used to treat migraine headache, tension headaches, cluster headaches, sinus headaches, hormonal headaches like menstrual migraine, and headaches due to
hypertension. Early research showed some promise, but conventional
medicine's bottom line was that there wasn't yet enough "evidence"
to justify recommending acupuncture as a first-line treatment. Now,
many well-designed studies have been completed and a systematic
review of 25 adult headache studies concluded that acupuncture *can*
provide relief superior to placebo, and superior even to some medications. In a total of seven trials involving 479 patients, on average 62%
had a significant positive response to acupuncture while only 45%
responded to medication.

A 2009 *Cochrane Review* reported the results of several large trials involving many thousands of patients. In the largest study, which
included patients with migraine, tension-type headache, and combination headache, those randomly assigned to receive acupuncture in
addition to routine care showed decreases in headache frequency and
pain intensity compared with patients assigned to routine care alone.
The 2009 *Cochrane Review* also looked at 22 trials involving only
migraine and concluded that acupuncture *consistently demonstrated
more benefit than routine care alone*, and may be more effective than

the preventive headache medication metoprolol (a beta-blocker) with significantly fewer side effects.

In studies looking at treatment for acute migraine, acupuncture performed similarly to the popular headache drug Imitrex (sumatriptan) although sumatriptan provided a faster response. Acupuncture has proven to be a viable nondrug treatment for patients with migraine headache and those with episodic tension-type headache, but is less effective for chronic tension headaches. Some case studies support its use in treating the facial pain disorder trigeminal neuralgia. We still don't know how acupuncture's pain-relieving effect works, but some research points to disruption in the communication of pain signals from the cranial blood vessels and the outermost layer of the meninges, or to the suppression of substance P, an inflammatory neurotransmitter.

All needles used in acupuncture must be single-use needles. When needles are correctly placed, there are few serious side effects associated with acupuncture. Occasional bleeding, pain at the insertion site, and aggravation of symptoms have been reported. People with skin infections, bleeding disorders, or those taking blood thinners should avoid acupuncture and it is not recommended for infants or young children. There are a few specific acupoints that should not be used on pregnant women.

BOTANICAL MEDICINE

Botanical medicine, or herbal medicine, uses a wide array of teas, tinctures, and topical applications to treat illness. Using herbal remedies may seem unscientific to some people, but many of our most useful medications were originally derived from plants, from simple aspirin, to chemotherapy drugs. In fact, it is very important for all of us to realize that herbal medicines are real medicines. They can have very powerful effects on the body and can interact with other drugs, which puts patients at risk for potential interactions from the following combinations:

Blood thinners: Always disclose to your health care provider any herbs, supplements, or teas that you use for your health. Failing to do so could cause a potentially serious problem if you were to undergo surgery, for example, because many herbs have blood-thinning properties. These herbs include the "four G's": ginger, garlic, *Ginkgo biloba*, and ginseng (*Panax ginseng* and *Siberian ginseng*). Patients who already take blood thinning drugs, like Coumadin (warfarin) need to be especially careful. Feverfew, a very popular herb in migraine prevention, can also increase the risk of bleeding and should not be taken before surgery or with NSAIDs like aspirin, ibuprofen, or naproxen.

Barbiturates: These drugs include Fioricet and drugs containing butalbital. These are sedating, and can be overly sedating when combined with sedating herbs like kava kava.

Calcium channel blockers: Used in migraine prevention, these drugs can interact with the herbs dong quai, guarana, and gingko, causing a variety of effects, including hypotension, or low blood pressure.

Antidepressants are commonly used in the treatment of many types of chronic pain as well as depression and can interact with the popular herb St. John's Wort. Taking St. John's wort with the tricyclic antidepressants amitriptyline, nortriptyline, doxepin, fluoxetine, and imipramine can lower the effective dose of these drugs in your system and should be avoided. Taking St. John's Wort with some anti-seizure medications may cause oversedation.

Dr. Christina Peterson, MD, a neurologist in Portland, Oregon, has written an overview entitled *Herbal Supplements and Medications: An Overview of Herb-herb and Drug-herb interactions* from which much of this information was drawn. See the website www.migraine-survival.com/herbal-supplements-and-medications-an-overview-of-herb-herb-and-drug-herb-interactions-2

What Nurses Know...

If you think you might be experiencing a hypersensitivity reaction or an interaction between your pharmaceutical drugs and an herbal preparation, contact your physician immediately. Many health provider groups have advice lines where you can reach a health professional any time. You can also report any adverse reactions to MedWatch, an FDA tracking program, at the following website: www.fda.gov/medwatch

Now that the warnings are out of the way, I'll let you in on some of my favorite herbal applications in headache treatment and prevention, and include information on any relevant studies. One of the easiest and most convenient ways to use herbal remedies is in a *topical application* applied to the skin. I've had modest results with St. John's wort oil applied to the tight muscles at the back of the head just where it meets the neck. And I particularly like a product called "Migrastick," a tiny roll-on vial of 100% natural essential oils of lavender and peppermint. It works best when applied at the *first twinge* of a migraine. Take care when applying to the forehead, a typical place for migraines to strike in women, because the oil may run down into and irritate the eye. It smells lovely, too, and it can be kept in your purse, car, or desk drawer. See the website www.migrastick.com/en/index.php

Butterbur (*Petasites hybridus*) has been used in Europe and more recently in the United States as a migraine preventive. It is thought to act as a calcium channel blocker, influencing the inflammatory cascade that precipitates a migraine. Butterbur must be prepared properly to remove toxins, so look for "Petadolex" or another product labeled "PA-free." Butterbur has done well in several studies, proving to be about twice as effective as placebo in decreasing the number of monthly migraine attacks. Butterbur can cause some mild digestive effects. It should not be used by pregnant women, but studies have shown it to be safe and effective in children and adolescents with migraine.

Feverfew (*Tanacetum parthenium*) has been used for hundreds of years to treat fever, arthritis, and headache. Feverfew is thought to inhibit platelet aggregation and decrease the inflammatory action of prostaglandins. Until recently, results in studies investigating feverfew in migraine prevention were inconsistent but its safety has not been a major issue. Standardizing the preparations for active parthenolide content and creating a more stable feverfew extract finally appears to have led to a significant outcome. In a study of 170 patients, a "clinically relevant" reduction in migraine frequency was reported in patients taking feverfew versus a placebo. More recently, researchers studying the benefits of feverfew developed a new application, combining the herb with ginger. The new product, called "LipiGesic-M," has proven to be safe and more effective than placebo in treating acute migraine, including the associated symptoms of nausea and vomiting, most likely due to the addition of ginger. It is currently available as a sublingual (under the tongue) lozenge, which, although well tolerated, caused some temporary mild numbness of the tongue. Feverfew should also not be used in pregnancy. It can cause uterine contractions resulting in miscarriage. It can also cause allergic reactions in people with hay fever, especially those also allergic to ragweed or chrysanthemums, to which feverfew is related.

Marijuana (*Cannabis sativa*) is now legalized for medicinal use in several states, and it has been suggested as a potential headache remedy. In fact, marijuana was often used for pain relief before

What Nurses Know...

CAN CHEWING SOME CELERY HELP YOUR HEADACHE?

Celery roots, leaves, stalks, and seeds have medicinal properties that may be beneficial for headache relief and prevention. Celery also provides a balanced profile of calcium, magnesium, potassium, and sodium—minerals the body needs. Studies show that celery contains several chemical compounds that help to relax and stabilize blood vessels, which may account for celery's apparent effectiveness in treating migraine headache, as well as its demonstrated ability to lower blood pressure. Some sources suggest chewing two to four stalks of cool, crisp celery at the first sign of a headache, or daily, to prevent headaches. Some migraine sufferers report success using 2 to 4 ounces of fresh celery juice flavored with a small amount of apple juice to stop a developing headache in 30 minutes or less. Celery seed is also used medicinally for headache prevention and treatment, although this remedy should NOT be used by pregnant women because it has been known to increase the risk of uterine contractions and could lead to miscarriage. Those using celery frequently should be careful to purchase only organic celery and wash it thoroughly before consuming.

pharmaceuticals were widely available. Substances found in cannabis may have the potential to reduce allodynia, to modulate pain, and to reduce nausea. Marijuana's efficacy in headache treatment has not yet been widely studied. But anecdotal reports and a few case studies have reported success in the treatment of chronic headaches, migraine, and cluster headache.

Black cohosh (*Actaea racemosa* or *Cimicifuga racemosa*) is interesting because it has the potential to both alleviate and cause headaches. It appears to be effective in helping to prevent menopausal migraines and other hormonally influenced headaches. Black cohosh contains fukinolic acid, an estrogen-like compound thought to be effective as a treatment for hot flashes, night sweats, and vaginal dryness but there is some evidence that it does not readily attach to estrogen receptors in the human body. Other components of the herb may contribute to its effectiveness, including some antiinflammatory and antispasmodic activity.

MayoClinic.com presents studies indicating black cohosh's effectiveness in treating menstrual migraines, possibly preventing headaches for up to six months. But the NIH reports that severe frontal headaches are also a common side effect of this powerful remedy, especially when it is taken in quantities exceeding the recommended dosage. "Remifemin" is a standardized product containing 20 mg of black cohosh per tablet and is usually taken twice daily.

Although widely used in Europe and popular with postmenopausal women, black cohosh should be used *with caution* until long-term studies can be completed, suggests The National Institutes of Health. The

What Nurses Know...

I highly recommend working with a qualified herbalist in your community if you wish to investigate other herbs that may be useful in treating headaches, including white willow bark (Salix alba), *peppermint (*Mentha piperita*), Passionflower* (Passiflora alata*), Blue Vervain (Verbena officinalis), and Catmint (*Nepeta sp.).*

NIH notes that adverse effects, although uncommon, have included gastrointestinal problems, dizziness, vision problems, and tremors. They also recommend that people suffering from liver disease, pregnant women, and those with a history of breast cancer avoid black cohosh.

Overall, botanical medicines are useful adjuncts to headache treatment and may be a good choice for patients who do not tolerate or desire to use pharmaceuticals. Interested readers can learn more about a variety of herbs and supplements at the National Institutes of Health's helpful website: http://ods.od.nih.gov/factsheets/list-all/

BIOFEEDBACK AND RELAXATION THERAPY

Biofeedback is a great technique for patients who cannot tolerate headache medications or who want to avoid medications during pregnancy. It may also be a good option for patients who have responded poorly to other treatments. In a typical biofeedback session, usually lasting 30 to 60 minutes, the therapist applies pads containing electrical sensors to the skin on different parts of the body. These sensors provide information about your skin temperature, heart rate, and muscle tension, and you can track changes in these parameters following visual cues like flashing lights or sound cues like different beeps.

Biofeedback therapy has been used for many decades to help patients gain control over specific physical symptoms, including pain, and to teach patients relaxation techniques. Biofeedback and relaxation therapy may also include teaching slow, relaxed abdominal (or diaphragmatic) breathing and positive visualization—like taking your mind to a quiet or happy place such as a sunny beach or quiet meadow. As you work on these relaxation techniques, you can immediately receive "feedback" on your physiological reactions. It is easy to see how pinpointing the tense muscles in your neck, and learning to consciously relax them, might reduce a tension headache. With practice you will be able to use these techniques on your own at home or at work without the biofeedback apparatus, which is a much more cost-effective option for patients in the long run. Although, this may sound very simple, biofeedback and relaxation techniques have proven their value in headache treatment, helping to reduce headache frequency by 45% to 60% for migraine headache and tension-type headache—roughly equivalent to the success rate of drugs like propranolol and amitriptyline. In a 2005 study, biofeedback-assisted diaphragmatic breathing and relaxation was only slightly more effective than propranolol in prevention of migraine headache over a 6-month period, but during the year following treatment, the patients who were taught biofeedback, breathing, and relaxation techniques had a much lower rate of headache reoccurrence: 9.4% versus 38.5% for the propranolol group. Chronic, severe headaches rarely respond to biofeedback alone, but this noninvasive therapeutic technique may be a useful coping tool when combined with other therapies, including preventive medications.

CHIROPRACTIC MEDICINE AND THE NUCCA TECHNIQUE

In essence, chiropractic medicine focuses on diagnosing and treating mechanical dysfunction in the musculoskeletal system, especially the spine. The principle hands-on technique is spinal manipulation to treat "subluxations," the misalignment of one or more vertebrae. But in recent years many chiropractors have taken on the role of promoting wellness, actively counseling patients on nutrition, exercise, and a healthy lifestyle.

If you tend to suffer most from cervicogenic or tension headaches, a chiropractic evaluation may be worthwhile. According to Dr. Stephanie Maj, 75% of her chiropractic patients have "head-forward posture," which can contribute to these kinds of headaches. Evaluating patients' sitting and standing posture should be an important part of chiropractic care, especially for patients complaining of headaches located at the base of the skull. A physical therapist can help you retrain your body to maintain proper posture to support the neck and head. Remember, "*Sternum up, and the head will follow.*"

However, a recent study on spinal manipulation suggested that although the practice was an effective headache treatment for patients with *cervicogenic headache* caused by neck strain, it was not superior in a study which compared it to sham or "made-up" treatment. The study's authors also feel that spinal manipulation holds significant risks for some patients, including increasing the possibility of transient ischemic attack, vertebral artery dissection and stroke. Many chiropractors disagree, and a recent *Cochrane Review* found spinal manipulation to be *"no more or less effective than medication for pain, physical therapy, exercises, ... or the care given by a general practitioner."*

NUCCA is a unique, much gentler and more precise form of cervical chiropractic adjustment advocated by an active educational organization called the *National Upper Cervical Chiropractic Association*, whose members focus their work on the relationship between the upper cervical spine and the central nervous system—including the brain stem. Carefully controlled contact on the first vertebrae in the neck (C-1) is designed to correct misalignment of the upper spine. The C-1 vertebrae, also called the Atlas, is a small ring-shaped bone located between the top of the spine and the base of the skull. NUCCA practitioners believe that correcting "Atlas Subluxation Complex Syndrome" has positive benefits on the nerves that control the body's vital functions, movement, sensation, and even behavior. I experienced periodic NUCCA sessions for chronic occipital neuralgia and felt it to be of significant value, but with these important cautions: The practitioner must have extraordinary skill, he or she must use the technique very carefully, and only in very specific situations involving misalignment of the C-1 vertebrae. To learn more about the NUCCA technique, see the website www.nucca.org/

CRANIOSACRAL THERAPY

Craniosacral therapy (CST) is a gentle hands-on technique that focuses on releasing restrictions in the tissues that surround the brain and spinal column—the central nervous system. The cranio-sacral system includes the specialized membranes and cerebrospinal fluid that surround and protect the brain and spinal cord. The cerebrospinal fluid pulses, in its own particular rhythm, up and down the spinal cord as it circulates around the brain tissue. Pioneered by a specialist in biomechanics, CST therapy is practiced by some physical therapists, massage therapists, and osteopathic physicians. It can be effective in treating upper back, neck, and head problems, including migraines and other headaches, chronic neck and back pain, and stress-related disorders.

EXERCISE

Exercise should be a way of life for all of us. But it isn't often recommended as a first-line treatment for headache prevention, so for many patients experiencing headaches, exercise might not immediately come to mind. However, exercise is well known to generate endorphins, our bodies' natural pain-reducing substances, and a few studies have shown positive benefits of aerobic exercise on reducing the frequency and intensity of migraine headache. A 2003 study followed 40 women with migraine headache for eight weeks and found that regular aerobic exercise decreased headache intensity, frequency, and duration. Brisk walking, cycling, swimming, jogging, cross-country skiing, and active dancing for 20 minutes or more are all great aerobic exercises. Working out at least three days a week is a good goal for most patients.

INTEGRATIVE MANUAL THERAPY

Integrative Manual Therapy, or IMT, is a powerful, yet noninvasive "health care process" practiced by some specially trained physical therapists, and it can be extremely effective in dealing with severe, persistent headaches. Using a gentle touch of the practitioner's hands, the technique works to re-establish normal rhythms in the body, to address pain and dysfunction, and to facilitate the body's ability to heal itself. (The cranio-sacral rhythm, discussed previously, is just one of the natural, ever-present rhythms in the body.) IMT builds on this foundation to work throughout the body's systems. See the Integrative Manual Therapy Association for more information: www.imtassociation.org/what-is-imt.asp

MASSAGE THERAPY, MYOFASCIAL RELEASE, AND TRIGGER POINT THERAPY

When you feel tense, your muscles are tight, and you feel a headache coming on, a massage sounds like just the ticket—but does it have any therapeutic value? Massage has many possible benefits for headache patients: It can enhance the relaxation response, help to increase blood flow to chronically tight muscles, reduce restrictions in tight tissues, and reduce the activity of trigger points. (Trigger points are small nodules of hyperactive contractile tissue within a muscle that are thought to play a role in generating and referring pain to the head.) According to some studies, massage is most helpful in treating tension-type headache. One small study followed patients who received twice-weekly massage sessions for four weeks. Therapists used a specialized protocol, including stretching and muscle energy techniques, to target six muscles of the head, neck and shoulder area: the upper trapezius, sternocleidomastoid, suboccipital, splenius capitis, levator scapulae, and temporalis muscles. The protocol also involved treating specific trigger points in the neck and shoulders. Compared with baseline levels, headache frequency was reduced after just the first week of massage and frequency continued to be reduced over the study period.

One of the special techniques massage therapists and physical therapists use is called myofascial release. Myofascial refers to "muscles" and "fascia"—a tough, elastic layer of tissue known as "fascia" covering the body's muscles, ligaments, tendons, and nerves. Under ideal circumstances, fascia helps to allow fluid movement of these various tissues against each other, while also forming a cushioning, protective sheath around each. Without their coating of fascia, many tissues, and especially nerves, would be subject to irritation caused by friction. Trauma, injury, and even lack of movement can cause these tissues to shrink, harden, and tighten, further limiting range of motion and inhibiting normal movement. Restricted fascia can sometimes cause nerve entrapment, resulting in chronic nerve irritation. Myofascial release is a specific type of therapy involving massage techniques that involve slowly stretching the involved tissues, freeing restrictions in the muscles and surrounding fascia. You can even learn to do this yourself in areas within your reach.

Some headache experts feel that many headache disorders may have an underlying myofascial cause and therapy aimed at reducing myofascial restrictions and keeping myofascial pain in check can prevent the occurrence of tension headaches and migraine. According to Dr. Stuart Stark, director of the Neurology and Headache Treatment Center in Alexandria, Virginia, "*Myofascial therapy, as well as massage and trigger point therapy (applying pressure to certain affected areas), may benefit patients with chronic tension-type headaches or chronic migraine headaches,*" with benefits lasting up to one month.

Hal S. Blatman, MD, states, "*Myofascial trigger points in the muscles of the scalp, jaw, neck, shoulders and upper back refer pain to the head and face.*" Dr. Blatman gives several specific examples: The sterno-cleidomastoid muscle refers pain to the forehead, sinus, ear, and back of the head; trigger points at the back of the skull can radiate pain to the back of the head, across the top of the skull, to the forehead–causing tension and migraine headache. We know that some patients respond well to therapies such as massage, myofascial release, and trigger point therapy. You can ask for referrals to health profession-als who practice these techniques, and be sure to report back to your physician about your progress.

MINDFULNESS-BASED STRESS REDUCTION

A specific program called Mindfulness-Based Stress Reduction (MBSR) has been used to alleviate pain and increase patients' feel-ing of well being. Weekly sessions teach "mindfulness," a practice of moment-to-moment awareness originally developed in the Buddhist tradition. MBSR allows continuous observation and acceptance of physical sensation, emotions, thoughts, and images but teaches patients to refrain from judgment and to avoid associating these feelings and thoughts with emotional value. Over time this process appears to reduce stress and to reduce the "stress hormone" cortisol. Practicing MBSR may be of value for people with physical and mental illness and for those who are chronically under high levels of stress. In helping to reduce stress, MBSR may be useful in preventing ten-sion-type headaches and migraine.

NATUROPATHIC MEDICINE

Portland, Oregon, is home to a number of schools of alternative medicine, including the National College of Naturopathic Medicine (NCNM)–the oldest accredited naturopathic medical school in North America. As a result, Portland may have more naturopaths, or NDs, than any other city in the United States. Naturopathic medicine has found its true place in health care as a complement to conventional medicine, focusing on prevention and wellness, as well as the treatment of some types of chronic illness. It has grown from a little-known field of natural medicine to a state-of-the-art, widely accepted, primary care and preventive medicine practice. It is important to understand that naturopathy is practiced by doctors who go to medical school for 4 to 5 years following their undergraduate curriculum. Naturopathic doctors are licensed to practice medicine in 11 U.S. states and 5 Canadian provinces. Many naturopathic physicians practice alongside medical doctors (MDs) and osteopathic doctors (DOs) in integrative health group practices. Drawing on many traditions from cultures around the world and using many different modalities of healing, naturopathic medicine is based on the following six principles:

- The body has an inherent ability to establish, maintain, and restore health; the physician's role is to facilitate and augment this process, identify and remove obstacles to recovery, and support health.
- Symptoms are expressions of the body's attempt to heal and are not the cause of disease. Underlying causes may be physical, emotional, and spiritual, and the physician must evaluate and direct treatment at underlying causes.
- Therapy should be complementary to the body's natural healing process, and there is a strong adherence to the principle: "First Do No Harm."
- The focus is on treating the whole person, which requires an individualized and comprehensive approach to diagnosis and treatment.
- The physician also acts as a teacher, playing a major role in educating and encouraging patients to make positive changes which support their health.
- The ultimate goal is prevention, accomplished through educating patients and promoting healthy lifestyle habits, with an emphasis on building health rather than fighting disease.

Naturopathic doctors may specialize in various areas of complementary medicine, such as botanical medicine, clinical nutrition, or obstetrics and midwifery.

OXYGEN THERAPY

Physicians often prescribe oxygen in emergency-room treatment of acute headaches like migraine. Short-term high-flow oxygen has also been observed in the clinical setting to help alleviate cluster headache, and now there is new research to further support its use. A recent study showed that treating cluster headache symptoms soon after onset with inhaled high-flow oxygen was more likely than placebo to result in pain relief after 15 minutes. Newer acute headache therapies may someday include the use of hyperbaric oxygen (HBOT), which administers 100% oxygen at pressures greater than 1 atmosphere of pressure, but at present hyperbaric oxygen carries higher risks and is not widely available.

PHYSICAL THERAPY

Physical therapists are experts in understanding how the body moves, how the many different parts of our musculoskeletal system interact, and how to correct physical problems that may contribute to headaches. Many headache patients suffer from chronic muscle tightness and discomfort, improper posture, and other musculoskeletal abnormalities. Therefore, physical therapy (PT) is often recommended for use in both migraine and tension headache, and may be especially effective in reducing frequency, intensity, and duration in chronic tension-type headache. PTs have a wealth of tools and techniques at their disposal, including teaching exercises and stretching routines, and coaching patients on ergonomics for home, work, and athletic activities. PT is not usually invasive or uncomfortable and over time you may come to enjoy a good working relationship with your therapist. Your doctor can write a prescription to "evaluate and treat" your headache condition and your therapist will take it from there, designing a personalized treatment plan. PT is covered by most types of health insurance.

VITAMINS AND OTHER SUPPLEMENTS

Many people take vitamins and "nutraceutical" supplements for health, but are there some that have a proven track record in helping prevent headaches? The five supplements with the best clinical evidence of effectiveness are magnesium, riboflavin (vitamin B2), coenzyme Q10, folic acid, and fish oil/Omega-3 fatty acids.

1. *Magnesium*: Several studies have shown that levels of magnesium measured in red blood cells, serum and brain tissue were

much lower in adults and children with migraines than in those who do not have migraines. Menstruation and stress, two factors common in triggering migraines, can deplete magnesium levels. And experimentally, it has been shown that magnesium deficiency can result in arterial spasm, spreading cortical depression, central neurotransmitter release, and increased clumping of platelets, each believed to play a role in the development of migraine.

Numerous studies have now shown magnesium supplementation to be a safe, effective way to reduce the frequency of migraines by close to 50%, a typical goal for a positive treatment response. Adverse effects are not serious and are usually limited to gastrointestinal irritation and/or diarrhea, especially if exceeding the recommended daily dose. Magnesium often comes in doses of 250 mg, which falls within the recommended dose of 100 to 300 mg twice daily. Some studies have investigated intravenous (IV) magnesium for treating acute migraine, but this is impractical for most patients. A middle ground may be the use of *sublingual* ionic magnesium drops or spray, which I have found to be very effective when taken at the first sign, or even during the aura period, of a migraine headache. An added benefit is that sublingual magnesium is very easy to adjust gradually drop by drop to achieve the desired effect. (It doesn't taste very good, but diluting it with a small amount of water helps.) Magnesium has a laxative effect and taking too much will likely result in a quick trip to the bathroom. This usually prevents magnesium overdose, but magnesium toxicity can occur, with symptoms including muscle weakness. Patients with kidney disease should not take supplemental magnesium unless directed by a physician.

2. *Riboflavin:* Also known as vitamin B2, riboflavin plays a role in mitochondrial energy production within the cells, which may account for its relationship to migraine headache. (Mitochondrial energy production is thought to be impaired in migraineurs.) Favorable studies have led to wider acceptance of riboflavin's role in reducing the frequency and severity of migraine. Dr. Alan Gaby, MD, has expressed the opinion that very high amounts of riboflavin are not necessary and that doses of 25 mg/day seem to be effective for most patients.

3. *Coenzyme Q10*: Coenzyme Q10 *also* plays an important role in mitochondrial energy production. In studies, supplementing with CoQ-10 has reduced headache *frequency* by greater than 50%, but had little effect on headache intensity or headache duration. The recommended dose for headache prophylaxis in adults is 60 to 300 mg/day. CoQ-10 is one of the most effective and popular treatments for migraine headache and abdominal migraine in children and adolescents. For additional information about the effectiveness of coenzyme Q10 (or CoQ-10) in headache prevention, see Chapter 8—Headaches in Children.

4. *Folic Acid and other B-vitamins:* Children with recurrent migraines were found, in one study, to have high levels of homocysteine, a well-recognized cause of inflammation in the body. High homocystemine levels have, in turn, been linked to *low* levels of folic acid. In a study on 16 children with migraines and high homocysteine levels, daily supplementation with 5 mg of folic acid led to a complete resolution of migraines in 10 children. Five of the remaining children experienced a 75% reduction in migraine frequency. Follow-up tests showed a normalization of homocysteine levels in all 16 patients. Migraine headache patients may want to have their homocysteine levels checked with a routine lab test. Patients with high homocysteine levels can make dietary changes, including eating more fruits and vegetables and may supplement with 5 mg/day of folic acid. Combining folic acid with vitamin B6 and vitamin B12 may also reduce the frequency and severity in adult migraine with aura. Vitamin B12 may play a role in migraine due to its ability to its interaction with nitric oxide.

5. *Fish oil/Omega-3 fatty acids:* For more than a decade we've heard about the benefits of Omega-3 fatty acids and other substances in fish oil, but is it also useful in preventing headaches? In double-blind studies, the results have sometimes been confusing because the "placebo"—olive oil—*also* was associated favorably with *significant reductions in migraine headache frequency.* Both olive oil and fish oil have antiinflammatory properties and perhaps *both* are helpful additions to a headache-prevention diet. But be sure to discuss taking them with your doctor: In addition

to its antiinflammatory effects, fish oil is known to have *blood thinning effects.*

Your Headache Toolkit—"Don't Leave Home Without It"

It is my sincere hope that frequent headaches do not disrupt your life. By building a trusted health care team and perhaps by incorporating some CAM therapies you should begin to make progress in managing your headaches. It also helps to have some practical tools to use when a headache strikes without warning, or when you're away from home. Consider choosing from the following:

- Instant coffee packets for helping to constrict blood vessels in migraine headache.
- Your usual OTC products or properly labeled prescription medications.
- An orthopedic neck pillow: Choose a soft pillow that still holds its shape or you may not enjoy using it.
- A flexible ice-pack shaped like a neck collar. I bought mine through my chiropractor's office. Applying a soft, flexible cold-pack is useful in migraine or tension headache, and can be very effective in helping to alleviate headaches localized at the base of the skull. Ice was a great benefit in helping me manage the pain of occipital neuralgia and I highly recommend it. Some patients like to alternate cold treatments with applications of warm, moist heat. A microwaveable soft rice-filled neck pillow also helps increase circulation and can help with neck and shoulder stiffness and tense muscles—very useful in tension headache.
- Warm, wool socks. Why? Many people with migraines report having very cold hands and feet during a migraine attack. Wearing socks may help to increase blood flow to the feet.
- Dark sunglasses: Always keep a pair in your car and in your purse.
- Lavender-peppermint oil in roll-on form; "Migrastick" is one brand.

- Herbal teas, in loose form or in bags; Alvita brand feverfew or peppermint are good choices. *Ashwagandha* or *linden* tea may be useful in stress-induced tension headache.

What Nurses Know...

Both warm and cool treatments should be well wrapped in soft towels before application to prevent harm to the skin, and be applied for a maximum of 20 minutes, followed by a rest period of at least 20 minutes (then repeat if desired after skin has returned to normal temperature). Never use a heat application while sleeping. For more tips on using warm and cold treatments to alleviate headache, I recommend reading chapter 10 in The TMJ Healing Plan *by physical therapist Cynthia Peterson.*

Tension-Type Headache

For several years I was working as a nurse-midwife in a large hospital in Germany where there seemed to be constant friction between the nurse-midwives and the obstetricians. At the end of each day as I was driving home I could feel extreme tension in my shoulders and neck. I could feel it creeping up the back of my head, the muscles clenching in a tight band that I knew would result in a bad headache. After a while I made the decision to quit my job. Fortunately, I soon found a wonderful opportunity to work with a group of like-minded nurse-midwives in a free-standing birth center, where we could conduct births the way we intuitively knew they should happen, in a more home-like setting, and allowing more time for the birth process to take place. Shortly after transforming my work environment, I noticed that the muscle tension was completely gone, and—NO MORE HEADACHES! SUSANNAH

Tension-type headache is the first of the *primary* headaches—the most common type of headaches we experience and the type of headaches most often seen by doctors and other health care providers.

The National Institute of Neurological Disorders and Stroke (NINDS) reports that more than 45 million Americans suffer from frequent or recurring headaches. A very large percentage of these are classified as tension-type headaches (TTH). Tension headaches also used to be called muscle contraction headaches.

Tension-Type Headache

Tension headaches are what most people think of as "regular headaches" or "just a headache," or even "a stress headache." Often described as a dull, aching pain radiating from either the forehead or back of the head, TTH can worsen to encompass the entire head. People also frequently complain that neck pain and tight neck muscles that precede or accompany the headache are persistent problems for them. There does not seem to be a clear physiological explanation for how tension headaches develop in all individuals and there may be various factors that combine to produce TTH, but overexertion, eyestrain, and myofascial pain often play a role in TTH. Some research has shown that muscle tension is permanently heightened in chronic tension headache patients and will continue to contribute to headache pain in the absence of rehabilitative therapies. Pain generated from muscular or myofascial tissues tends to have characteristics similar to tension headache pain—dull, achy, radiating, and diffuse.

Tension frequently builds up in the muscles and surrounding fascia of the upper back, shoulders, neck, and jaw, and in the smaller muscles surrounding the head. Contributing factors include ergonomically incorrect work routines and clenching or grinding one's teeth as a result of stress. But a significant cause is postures which chronically strain the neck muscles that support the head and allow the head to bend, or droop, forward. Chronically tipping the head forward to look at computer screens, visual displays of smartphones, sewing, or crafts can lead to a buildup of unhealthy muscle tension, causing cervicogenic headache, a disorder which can overlap with TTH. The head-forward position also compresses the C-1 and C-2 vertebrae, putting pressure on the associated nerves. Due to this nerve irritation, right-sided upper neck pain and stiffness generally refer pain to the right side of the head, and left-sided upper neck pain and stiffness refer pain to the left side. If your tension headaches originate in the upper cervical spine, techniques designed to help you restore normal movement and alleviate pressure on these nerves can help to alleviate tension headaches.

WHO GETS THEM AND WHY?

Tension headaches, also called tension-type headaches (TTH), are the most common headache type, affecting 78% of the general population, and about 3% of the population suffers from chronic tension headaches. TTH occurs in episodes, or attacks, which can be frequent or infrequent. This type of "episodic" TTH is the most common headache disorder worldwide. Unfortunately, TTH can also occur very often, and if present on at least 15 days per month they are classified as chronic tension-type headache (CTTH). CTTH is far more disabling than occasional tension headache episodes.

TTH affects slightly more women than men, and begins to affect people in their teens and early twenties. And it is my belief that TTH is also common but may be misdiagnosed in younger children due to their inability to articulate what they are feeling. TTH in very young children may be perceived by parents as simply a change in behavior, such as withdrawing from activities, or an escalation in fretfulness resulting in a "meltdown." (See Chapter 8.)

Certainly stress seems to be one of the most important factors in tension headaches, as you can see from Susannah's story, and it is also typical that the headache ends when the stress that brings on the headaches ceases to be a problem. Consistent with many other headache types, family history of tension headaches is also predictive and is present in about 40% of patients.

SYMPTOMS

People often describe a band of constriction, pressure, and pain surrounding the head. The pain is not located on one side, as it usually is in migraine and cluster headaches, but affects both sides of the head. TTH differs from migraine in other ways as well—the pain rarely worsens with physical exertion or position changes and it is not usually accompanied by the nausea and sensory changes common in migraine headache. But sometimes, some people do have the

What Nurses Know…

UNDERSTANDING SIGNS & SYMPTOMS

Throughout the book I use the words "signs" and "symptoms" when discussing headache types. It is helpful to know that "signs" refer to objective observations which your nurse or doctor is able to hear, see, feel, or measure, as well as test results. "Symptoms" are subjective—things that you, can feel, see, hear, or experience using other senses. There can be some overlap between signs and symptoms. You feel itchy—a symptom, but you also have a visible rash—a sign your doctor can observe. Pain is an important subjective symptom which can only be felt by the individual. Objective signs of pain include elevated pulse and blood pressure, as well as facial grimacing. You may feel feverish, a subjective symptom, and a thermometer also indicates that you have a high temperature, an objective sign. Or you may feel shaky, sweaty or flushed—observations your nurse or doctor is also able to notice.

sensitivity to light common to migraines. Tension headaches can last from less than an hour to several days and may be preceded by a single stressful event, or may result from the accumulated daily stresses of driving, working, and multi-tasking in other areas of one's life. People with mild to moderate TTH are usually able to continue with normal routines.

DIAGNOSIS

There are no tests to diagnose TTH. Diagnosis is based on an individual's history of the headache pattern and symptoms, and it must exclude other possible headache diagnoses. Although TTH usually affects both sides of the head, in special cases generally associated with poor posture or other musculoskeletal causes, tension headaches can sometimes be unilateral. A symptom that doctors look for to confirm tension headache is tenderness at the base of the skull or back of the neck, signs that these muscles are strained and inflamed. This sensation is really more of an actual soreness rather than heightened skin sensitivity found in migraine.

TTH can occur along with other headache disorders and can be a part of a "combination headache" or "mixed headache". Similarly, when a person experiencing migraines begins to also have the type of chronic daily muscle tension common to patients with frequent tension-type headaches, they may also be said to suffer from mixed tension-migraine headaches. And in some people, ignoring a tension headache, or suffering a treatment-resistant headache, seems to be a trigger for also developing a migraine later in the day. Treat your tension headaches early, and you might be able to avoid developing a really entrenched headache that lasts for days, or even a migraine, which often includes other unpleasant symptoms. Some authorities consider TTH and migraine to share a single cause, and the research is ongoing.

I have been challenged by tension headaches most of my life. The first one, when I was about eight years old, was bad enough for me to remember. By nightfall it was so bad I was biting on my sheets and begging my parents for help. When these happened my dad would often press my head between his hands firmly to equalize the pressure in my head, ease the tension, or some combination of both; I don't really know why his strange remedy helped, but it did. In the 1970s, we didn't really have pediatric pain relievers that I can remember. My tension headaches start in my shoulders and creep up the back of my neck into my head where, if not managed soon enough, they can get so bad I become nauseated.

—LOUISE

TREATMENT

Many people associate the class of headache medications called "triptans", including the popular drugs Imitrex and Maxalt, with migraine exclusively, but there is some evidence that these serotonin-agonists are effective in treating TTH too, although to a slightly lesser degree than their effectiveness in treating migraine. (See Chapter 7.) However, over-the-counter analgesics are the medications most often used to treat TTH. These include both various forms of acetaminophen (Tylenol,

Paracetamol), and the nonsteroidal antiinflammatory drugs (NSAIDs), which include analgesics like aspirin, ibuprofen (Advil), and naproxen (Naprosyn, Alleve). It is very important to avoid exceeding the recommended dose of these widely-available over-the-counter (OTC) drugs and to follow manufacturer's instructions regarding food and drink. In particular, NSAIDs must never be taken on an empty stomach, because even when taken as directed, all NSAIDs have the potential to cause gastric irritation and injury to the intestinal mucosal lining. Some patients with TTH respond well to cold, caffeinated drinks or medications containing a moderate amount of caffeine.

What Nurses Know...

A 2011 study in the British Medical Journal *suggests that NSAIDs may be linked to a 40% increased risk of heart arrhythmias such as atrial fibrillation or atrial flutter. If severe, these irregular heart rhythms can allow blood clots to form in the heart, increasing the risk of strokes. Aspirin is also an NSAID but does not appear to carry the same risk as ibuprofen and naproxen. Tylenol is not an NSAID as it does not decrease inflammation, but overuse may lead to toxicity and liver damage.*

I am not trying to be alarmist, but as a nurse I am concerned about the very casual use and overuse of these medications in all age-groups, worldwide. I believe that we would do well to remember, or, in the case of young people, to learn some of the non-drug comfort measures commonly in use before these medications were available. I highly recommend topical treatments like appropriately-applied medicated patches, massage, heat, and ice, as well as regular exercise and relaxation exercises to reduce muscle tension. We need to return to these older, reliable comfort treatments instead of always relying on not-so-harmless medications. We also need to take responsibility for caring for our bodies, reducing stress, and avoiding our individual headache triggers.

For persistent or severe TTH, doctors sometimes combine analgesics with other medications, including butalbital (isometheptene mucate), an intermediate-acting barbiturate. Fioricet, a prescription medication combining butalbital, acetaminophen, and caffeine, is sometimes used to treat tension headaches. But patients must take care not to use these medications more frequently than necessary, as doing so may actually create more headaches: These types of medications can increase the frequency of TTH and can lead to addiction and medication overuse headache. If you are using analgesics to treat your headaches more often than two or three times per week, you could be at risk for *medication-overuse headache* (MOH). This does not mean that your headache pain should be *ignored*, but that you should discuss with your physician other alternatives, including adjustments in lifestyle, exercise, diet, and stress, tobacco use, and, in many cases, the addition of a preventive medication can be very effective.

Physical therapy is *very* useful in treating tension headaches, and a variety of techniques may be used, including a muscle energy technique to help return the cervical joints to proper alignment and alleviate pressure on the nerves that send pain to the head. (This gentle, sustained, technique bears no relationship to chiropractic manipulation.) A physical therapist can also assess your musculoskeletal system and posture, and provide exercises that may help you prevent a buildup of muscle tension. You can ask your doctor for a referral for physical therapy evaluation and treatment. Massage is also a very useful therapy for episodic tension headache. One study found massage to be helpful in reducing frequency, intensity, and duration of headaches, increasing range of motion in the neck, and decreasing medication use. Acupuncture may also be helpful in treating TTH, although the evidence isn't as clear as it is with migraine headache.

PREVENTION

You may benefit from an evaluation by other health care practitioners, including an ergonomic specialist to look at your work station, but working on reducing stress may yield the best results when it comes to TTH.

Prevention is a worthy goal, especially in the case of chronic health issues. Preventive medications are sometimes used to decrease the frequency and severity of TTH, or to prevent the development of chronic TTH. These can include amitriptyline (Elavil), nortriptyline, doxepin, and fluoxetine (Paxil). These drugs are mainly known as antidepressants, but they are often used as an adjunct in chronic pain treatment. Antidepressant medications should begin at a low dose, and be increased slowly while monitoring for side effects, which may include dry mouth, drowsiness, foggy thinking, constipation, weight gain, and changes in libido.

Every medication has side effects, both short term and long term. Remember to discuss all medication side effects with your physician and pharmacist. Response to medications is highly individualized, and there are often alternatives that work well with fewer side effects. Be sure to review all of the nondrug approaches suggested in the previous chapters, including making appropriate lifestyle changes. Your body will thank you!

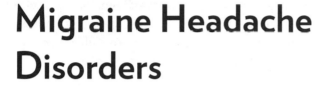

Migraine Headache Disorders

After many Board meetings it's as though somebody unplugs a cork in the side of my head—except instead of letting things out it seems to let things in. At other times, the pain begins around my head rather than in my head—then it fills my head and goes down into my gut, and from there into every part of my body so that my headache is a full-blown migraine. The nausea begins and the pain around my head is intense. I cannot eat or talk to anyone, and I have to dim the lights—if not lie in the dark. Oddly the relief of a stressful event somehow comes in the form of a migraine attack. I try to avoid caffeine and triggers like chocolate. But in the end, like a mountain lion, a bad headache can strike at any time, with no rhyme or reason.   AARON

Migraine: Not Just Another Headache

Most of us know that a migraine is not just a run of the mill headache, that it may be more severe, and even that there may be other associated symptoms. Most of us also know someone who suffers from migraines, because nearly 28 million Americans do. Migraine is the primary headache disorder most often seen by neurologists and is more variable than other primary headaches.

Migraine sufferers, or "migraineurs," come from both genders and from all backgrounds. Members, past and present, of this vast group include: poet Emily Dickinson, author Joan Didion, entertainer Elvis Presley, and Cindy McCain—a stroke-survivor and migraine health-care advocate. Migraine has a huge impact on health and healthcare—of all the headache types, migraine stands out as the most expensive to treat. Cluster headache may be more painful and tension headache more common, but migraine has the distinction of causing the most severe pain in the largest number of people overall. In addition, many people develop daily or near-daily chronic migraines, greatly affecting their quality of life.

There are two main forms: migraine without aura, and the less common migraine with aura—which includes sensory disturbances such as visual distortions. Migraine with aura has recently been linked to an increased risk of ischemic stroke, especially in women. Migraine has also been linked with a number of other disorders, including epilepsy, panic disorder, asthma, and depression. People who suffer from migraines are almost six times more likely to also suffer from depression, and those who suffer from depression are more than three times as likely to develop migraines. Before looking at typical symptoms, standard diagnosis, and options for treatment, let's learn more about the causes and complications of this disorder.

What Causes Migraine?

It is now widely accepted that migraine headache is a biological disorder that originates deep in the brain, and that the primary mechanism is abnormal hyperexcitability of nerve cells triggered by the brain's reaction to an event that overstimulates the senses. It is thought that this hypersensitivity is an inherited abnormality caused by the body's response to the activity of neurotransmitters like serotonin and glutamate, which play a role in migraine. Research in genetics has already located at least one genetic marker identified with a predisposition to migraines, a gene variant associated with the metabolism of glutamate—which is the most abundant "excitatory" neurotransmitter in our bodies and strongly suspected to be involved with the auras associated with migraine. There may be several different abnormal genes involved in migraine, which may account for differences in symptoms. Simply put, the brains of people who experience migraines are more sensitive to ordinary stimuli—so perhaps it isn't surprising that so many artists, writers, and entertainers suffer from migraine headaches.

More specifically, migraine is a "brain disorder," characterized by repeated attacks of cortical spreading depression—CSD (or alternately, spreading depression)—which cause the curious symptoms of migraine headache disorders. CSD refers to a series of rapid changes in the electrical charge of nerve cells, causing a sudden wave of temporarily increased blood flow across the brain and brain stem. In some cases, the arteries in the brain temporarily expand by more than 50%, providing oxygen-rich blood to adjacent brain tissues. Even so, during a migraine attack, blood flow in the brain is erratic and areas of the brain farthest from oxygen-rich blood vessels can receive too little blood flow, leading to physical damage to individual nerve cells. The wave of heightened nerve cell activity is followed by a period of suppressed nerve cell activity, and a corresponding rapid but longer lasting decrease in blood flow across the brain. But, as seen in imaging studies, the period of suddenly increased—then decreased—blood flow in the brain does not coincide with the pain or severity of migraine. So, what does cause the pain of migraine? Some brain scientists believe the pain actually originates outside the brain, in the superficial temporal arteries which branch off the external carotid arteries that supply blood to the head, neck, and face (Figure 7.1).

The superficial temporal arteries consist of two major vessels—the frontal branch running from about the inside of the earlobe, across the temples to the forehead and brow region, and the parietal branch, which curves around the top of the ear and supplies blood to the top of the head.

Smaller vessels branch off from these to supply blood to the face, jaw, and back of the head. The intensity of migraine pain is closely related to the force of pulsations in these arteries, which corresponds to an increase in blood vessel diameter on the affected side of the head. What causes this blood vessel dilation? Research points

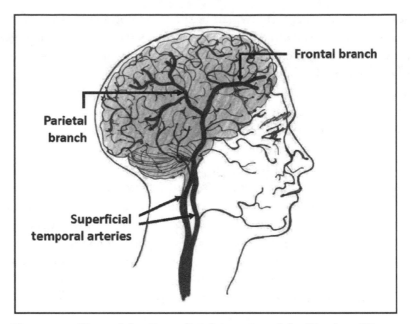

Frontal branch

Parietal branch

Superficial temporal arteries

Figure 7.1 View of the Superficial Arteries of the Head and Face

to a powerful vasodilator known as "calcitonin gene-related peptide" (CGRP). Imaging studies have shown significant differences in the blood flow in these superficial arteries, when migraineurs are experiencing headaches:

- During migraine headache, blood flow on the painful side is greater than on the unaffected side, and is also increased over levels in nonheadache subjects.
- Vasoconstricting medications causes measurable decreases in blood flow and can reduce a migraine.
- Similarly, triptan medications have reduced CGRP levels in migraine headache pain.

Migraine-provoking agents tend to cause blood vessel dilation, or expansion, and effective medications used to treat acute migraine usually cause blood vessel constriction, or narrowing. The newest drugs proposed to treat migraine (see Chapter 17) help to prevent CGRP's vasodilating effect on the superficial temporal arteries.

Other factors suspected to be involved in the development and unfolding of a migraine headache include central nervous system sensitivity that leads to lowered pain threshold and localized neu-rogenic inflammation. Localized neurogenic inflammation is a type of inflammation that is generated by the nervous system, instead of in response to trauma or infection. The ability to block neurogenic inflammation is one reason why drugs like triptans (Imitrex, Maxalt) are effective in stopping the pain of migraine headache.

Who Gets Them and Why?

Like some other primary headache types, migraine headaches tend to have a strong familial tendency—at least half of migraineurs have a family member who also suffers from this disorder. Most sources agree that migraines in adults are more than twice as common in women—affecting roughly 7% to 8% of men and 17% to 18% of women. Migraines affect a quarter of American women at some point in their lives, and migraine headache patterns and forms can change through-out the lifespan (learn more in Chapter 9).

Symptoms

Beyond the painful, one-sided, characteristic headache, migraines are accompanied by a host of other symptoms that may occur well before, immediately prior to, during, and after the attack. The four phases of a migraine are:

- Prodrome
- Aura
- Headache
- Postdrome

Related terms include prodromal, referring to symptoms or events preceding the headache, and postdromal, referring to events or symp-toms following the resolution of the headache. In some migraineurs these four features are quite distinct, but in others they are not so clearly defined and not all patients experience all four phases of migraine each and every time. In fact, the majority of migraineurs never experience aura, for example. Migraine without aura is much more prevalent than migraine with aura. Symptoms of each phase of migraine are discussed below:

THE PRODROME

The prodrome (prodromal phase or "preheadache") is the period preceding the headache, when patients typically begin to experience some warning symptoms such as a deflated feeling, irritability, fatigue, and sometimes cravings for certain foods. Tight, sore, or stiff neck, vague nausea, temperature changes, and dizziness may also be present. The prodrome does not affect all migraineurs, but those who do experience such symptoms in the hours or days before a migraine can take preventive medications or avoid activities that would aggravate a headache.

THE AURA

An aura is a physical or sensory experience occurring in the hour or so immediately preceding headache. Typically it ranges from about 5 to 45 minutes prior to the headache. Auras can include transient visual changes, temperature changes, weakness, dizziness, nausea, and tingling or numbness in the hands, forearms, or face. Some frightening symptoms include confusion, vertigo (a sensation that the environment around you is spinning), and less commonly, even partial paralysis. However, changes in hearing, vision, and sensation are the most common in the roughly 20% of migraineurs who experience aura. Visual auras often include flashing or bright lights, blurred vision, or visual distortions that resemble looking through falling snow, a kaleidoscope, or a prism—but remember, not all auras are visual. A range of symptoms found in aura is illustrated in the four scenarios below:

> *Minutes before my migraines strike, I see a bright spot in my right eye, as if I've stared at the sun too long. This is followed by pain behind my right eye, stuffiness in my right nostril, and a feeling like I need to go lie down, then the throbbing headache begins in my right temple.*
>
> —ALLYSSA

> *My symptoms are very striking. I get a visual blind spot in the center of one eye. This can last for up to 20 minutes or so, then I get a series of bright sparks that move around like fireflies, and*

then my energy starts to drop quickly. I know a headache will not be long in following.

—ROB

About 45 minutes before a migraine hits like a sledge-hammer, I start to get a whooshing sound in my ear on the same side as the migraine. It isn't the same as hearing my pulse pound when I run too fast, just a consistent "whoosh" in time with my pulse. Although no pain is involved, it goes on for a very long time—at least until the headache begins, and sometimes it persists after. Sometimes there is a very mild ringing in the ear, like a high-pitched whine almost beyond hearing. My eye on that side will be mildly blurry, as if I need to rub it to clear it, but it doesn't clear. I get very tired and my hands get very cold. All of these sensations continue during the early part of the headache and slowly fade away. I know my headache is getting better when my hands start to warm up. But if my hands get very cold, I know it will be a very bad headache.

—ALICE

When I was a child my aura consisted of seeing bright orange and green moving swirls—colors that were very jarring and didn't belong together—like a scary, giant lollipop. As a child, it took some time for me to associate this affect, which was "visible" even behind my closed eyelids, with the headache that came later. I remember that having a high fever was a consistent trigger for developing this kind of visual aura followed by a bad headache.

—REBEKKAH

THE HEADACHE

We all know what a headache feels like, but in migraine, a headache is typically one-sided, very intense, and debilitating. It is usually difficult to function with a full-blown migraine. Clinically, the headache phase is also divided into early, middle, and late headache—which may be important to readers in understanding the treatment recommendations: For most people, treating with rescue medications early in the headache is more successful than treating in later stages after the headache is fully underway. By clinical definition, symptoms of migraine headache typically include: nausea and/or vomiting, sensitivity to light and/or sound, anxiety, dizziness, and cognitive problems such as difficulty putting thoughts or words together coherently, slower recall of information, and slowed reflexes. Migraines frequently (but not always) strike in the early morning hours and an attack lasts from one to 72 hours, but migraine forms and patterns are variable.

However, most migraine headaches last at least four hours, and a key feature is pain that is worsened by physical activity. The body may experience temperature fluctuations, with hot flashes, chills, or lack of normal blood flow to extremities. Raynaud's syndrome, which results in painfully cold hands and feet, is common in migraineurs. Some people with migraine headache can have accompanying nasal congestion or a runny nose, usually on the same side as the headache. Migraine may include activation of the body's sympathetic nervous system—which controls our "fight-or-flight" responses. Increased sympathetic nervous system activity may cause the associated intestinal symptoms such as nausea, vomiting, and diarrhea, as well as delay absorption of oral medications. Our fight-or-flight response also decreases blood flow to the extremities, leading to a pale face and cool hands and feet.

THE POSTDROME

Following a migraine, there is a "postdromal period," during which patients describe feeling fatigued, foggy-headed, and even weak. Some patients will say, "My headache is gone, but I feel like I've been run over by a truck. I just want to go sleep it off." But some patients experience feelings such as profound relief or even euphoria. Sometimes this postdromal or "postheadache" period only lasts a few hours, but in some people it can last 24 hours. This corresponds to the period of abnormal cerebral blood flow that continues for up to 24 hours after a migraine headache. This is the "recovery period," during which you may find your reactions are slower and your word recall a little sluggish. Your energy level may take some time to return to normal. Take it easy and rely on your family or others to pick up the slack for a day or so, as you will most likely not be at your peak, mentally or physically—and you may also want to avoid making important decisions until you recover completely.

What Nurses Know...

PLAYING IT SAFE WHEN A SUDDEN HEADACHE STRIKES

All people who get migraines need to learn to recognize an aura or prodrome so they can pull off the road before vision, reflexes, or coordination become impaired. Carry a cell phone, bottled water, and medication, and always keep a pair of dark sunglasses in the car. If you work around or operate machinery, be cautious when you begin to feel that something "isn't quite right," or an aura may be developing. Take a break and get to a safe place to further assess your condition. If you are experiencing symptoms that interfere with your work, your safety, or the safety of others, inform your supervisor and DO NOT continue to work. Accidents can and do happen for exactly this reason. Just imagine an air traffic controller, train engineer, or heavy crane operator attempting to work with the blurred vision, sparkly or flashing lights, spots, or other visual changes accompanying or preceding a migraine! Know your individual pattern of symptoms and always put safety first.

Sensitivity to Light and Sound and Other Sensory Symptoms

Beyond headache pain, a group of symptoms associated with migraine headache disorders involves "sensory amplification." Sensitivity to light (photophobia) is a very common symptom associated with migraine, but it is not specific and occurs also in meningitis and some other conditions. Phonophobia is often used to mean sensitivity to sound, but it actually means "fear of sound." While loud noises can irritate many people, some migraineurs experience "hyperacusis," or an inability to tolerate ordinary sounds in the normal hearing range. When in the throes of a migraine, these background noises sound unpleasantly loud. Sometimes accompanied by tinnitus (ringing in the ears), this heightened sensitivity may be due to an abnormality in the way the nervous system processes sound. My sons have called this curious symptom of my migraines "super-hearing." When associated with migraine headache, hyperacusis and other sensory amplification usually recede once the migraine resolves. Hyperacusis can be a prodromal symptom, can be part of the aura, or can persist during the headache.

HEIGHTENED SENSE OF SMELL

One other symptom of sensory amplification is a heightened sense of smell (hyperosmia) or an aversion to smells (osmophobia), reported by many people to occur just before or during a migraine. People may also have an altered sense of taste and increased nausea with certain smells. Many patients have reported that strong scents often trigger migraine attacks. The most disturbing odors tend to be perfumes, aftershave cologne, cigarette smoke, scented soaps, and pungent foods. I experienced a heightened sense of smell for the 2 years during which I suffered from occipital neuralgia. From as far away as a dozen feet, I could uncannily tell my husband what he ate for lunch when he arrived home from work. This strange phenomenon disappeared when the neuralgia resolved and has never returned.

HEIGHTENED SENSE OF TOUCH

Allodynia exists when patients experience pain or discomfort from ordinary touch or pressure to the skin. People who suffer from allodynia during a migraine or as part of a chronic condition experience real pain from light touch, the brush of clothing, or simply the feeling of a breeze lifting their hair. Allodynia is another part of the sensory amplification picture caused by central nervous system sensitization, and it affects at least 63% of those with migraine headache, as well as people with some other neurological conditions. Women are more likely than men to suffer from cutaneous allodynia, and those who have higher headache frequency or chronic migraine, obesity, and depression are at greater risk. Allodynia is often a sign that the migraine is well underway, and the window of opportunity to effectively treat the headache with an acute medication is narrowing.

Usually sensation returns to normal following the migraine episode. It has been suggested that cutaneous allodynia is a risk factor for worsening migraine headaches and that patients with this neurological disorder may need to be treated more aggressively.

Diagnosis

Finding solutions to suspected migraine headache involves a visit to your primary care practitioner, who will conduct a thorough physical and neurological exam and ask you questions about your headache symptoms, duration, frequency, and severity. You can help by keeping an accurate headache diary and by describing your individual headache pattern. Be sure to mention any symptoms of an aura or prodrome and any possible headache triggers such as strong scents like cigarette smoke, drinking red wine, or eating chocolate. It is very helpful to know your family medical history—especially whether any member of your family has previously suffered from migraine headaches, which have a strong genetic component.

The International Classification of Headache Disorders-II (ICHD-II) has specific diagnostic criteria for migraine which will help your doctor to confirm the diagnosis, but another easy-to-use tool is "ID Migraine," a set of three simple questions. While suffering from a headache episode, do you have:

- Nausea
- Sensitivity to light
- "Disability" (the inability to carry out regular activities)

These three questions have proven to be good predictors of migraine and they can help to rule out sinus or tension headache, with which migraine is sometimes confused. For example, migraines can include nasal stuffiness or a runny nose as well as pain around the eye or in the forehead where sinus pain also commonly occurs. Similarly, migraine patients can have neck pain as part of their headache pattern, although pain and tension in the neck are usually associated with tension headache. But neither tension nor sinus headache are typically associated with sensitivity to light or nausea, and people with tension and sinus headaches are often able to carry on with work or social activities, while the migraine patient is effectively incapacitated. All of these variations in symptoms can be quickly addressed using the three-question ID-Migraine tool. Another tool, MIDAS (Migraine Disability Assessment), is used clinically to quantify a patient's headache disability based on loss of work days or school attendance during a 3-month period.

Response to headache treatment cannot reliably be used to diagnose migraine: Serotonin-agonist medications like triptans have also proven effective in treating other headache types, while some migraines have proven to be resistant to treatment with triptans.

Treatment

It is important to treat migraines during the early stages of the headache, or if you experience headache with aura, just before headache onset. Most patients desire to use, and need, a "rescue medication" for acute migraine in order to avoid disability and continue with life's responsibilities. Without a rescue medication, a migraine headache can be incapacitating, sometimes lasting for days.

Early rescue medications included the vasoconstricting ergot-derived drugs, or drugs combining caffeine with analgesics. Newer rescue medications include serotonin-agonist drugs like triptans that work by helping to shrink inflamed blood vessels which press on sensitive nerves. They have been life-changing for many headache patients. Medication types are grouped below:

- There are, at present, seven different triptans, and one triptan/ nonsteroidal antiinflammatory drug (NSAID) combination. Maxalt (rizatriptan) and Zomig (zolmitriptan) are available in a melt-away or ODT (oral dissolving tablet) which may be convenient when a headache comes on suddenly and the person does not have access to water. Other triptans are available in an oral tablet, and Imitrex (sumatriptan) is also available by self-injection. Research into a through-the-skin delivery systems for triptans continues, for obvious reasons: When a patient has severe nausea and vomiting with migraine it may be impossible to take an oral medication. Triptans revolutionized medical treatment of migraine headache through their effectiveness, high patient tolerance, and low rate of side effects. My own headaches responded very well to the

What Nurses Know...

Most migraine patients find that it really does help to pay attention and learn to recognize individual headache triggers, and then to make every effort to avoid them. Some well-known headache triggers are listed below:

- Bright or flashing lights—from an oncoming car hood or windshield, the flickering from a fluorescent light bulb, or possibly worst, a strobe light. Be sure to have a pair of sunglasses with you in your vehicle or purse, and try to avoid situations where a strobe light may be found. (Strobe lights have also been implicated in triggering seizures.)
- Emotional stress or physical stress in the form of overexertion can trigger an attack. You will need to find healthy ways to avoid stressful situations and to manage personal stress.
- Hormonal fluctuations tied to menstrual cycles, and to changes that occur during peri-menopause and menopause, can trigger migraines. This is often associated with dropping levels of estrogen. Speak with your physician about ways to minimize the effect of hormonal fluctuations on your headaches.
- Some specific foods have gained the reputation of being migraine triggers. These often include aged foods, alcohol, caffeine, and food additives such as MSG (monosodium glutamate).
- Low magnesium. In The Neurological Basis of Pain, Marco Papagallo writes, "It's estimated that 50% of patients with an acute migraine attack have lower magnesium levels than controls. Magnesium regulates a variety of receptor and neurotransmitter activity including substance P, nitric oxide, and serotonin. Multiples studies have shown systemic magnesium deficiency."

triptan rizatriptan (Maxalt). But, even these remarkable medications and other acute rescue medications may, if used more than 2 days per week, may place patients at risk for medication overuse headache (MOH)—also called "rebound headache"— although the relationship is certainly not as clear as with opioid medications. However, the true potential of triptans may not have yet been reached, as some physicians still prescribe alternate treatments first, before trying triptans. At least in the case of opiates, this isn't a very good idea, as seven separate studies of the triptan Maxalt (rizatriptan) showed that migraine patients who first used opioid medications had a less favorable response to triptans than those who did not. The study's outcome prompted the authors to suggest using triptans, rather than opioid narcotics, as a first-line acute migraine treatment. In fact, a study released in 2010 showed that although more people than ever are being treated for migraine, they are not always prescribed the most appropriate drugs. Instead of being offered newer "migraine-specific" medications, more general analgesics, including opioids, NSAIDs, and muscle relaxants are often used.

- An exciting new option for acute migraine treatment is a sublingual lozenge called LipiGesic-M, a combination of feverfew and ginger that has proven, in a placebo-controlled pilot study, to be safe and effective in aborting migraine headache and treating the associated symptom of nausea. Side effects included temporary oral numbness, but overall the feverfew/ginger preparation was well tolerated.

- Narcotic analgesics are not the best choice for management of migraine headache. They are addictive, carry significant side effects, and hold the greatest risk for causing medication overuse headache. All patients should strictly limit their use of narcotic analgesics to a maximum of 10 days per month. Even low-level use of these drugs decreases patients' responsiveness to other migraine medications. In most cases, your doctor can provide you with better options, although a narcotic may be used for an occasional migraine that falls outside of your monthly limit of triptans or for a particularly intractable migraine headache episode. The medication Stadol NS, a nonvasoconstricting abortive medication, is available by self-administered injection and in a nasal spray.

If you and your doctor decide that these medications are useful as part of your overall migraine management plan, it is important to follow a few precautions: All short-acting narcotics are sedating and are dangerous when combined with other sedating drugs or alcohol, all short-acting narcotics hold a potential for addiction, and using these drugs causes impairment—preventing safe driving or operating of machinery.

- Another medication sometimes used to treat migraines is Butalbital, an intermediate-duration barbiturate pain-reliever sometimes used in combination with acetaminophen and caffeine in the medication Fioricet. (An alternative is Fiorinal—a combination of Butalbital, aspirin, and caffeine.) Side effects of butalbital can include, at a minimum, dizziness, drowsiness, sedation, a feeling of intoxication, and nausea. Barbiturates are physically and psychologically addictive. They should never be mixed with alcohol, benzodiazepines (such as Valium), or narcotics (such as opioid pain relievers). Butalbital-containing medications can help to moderate the pain of a migraine attack, but cannot end the attack, and are not considered true "abortive" medications.

- In the past, an Emergency Department visit for a migraine headache usually involved injection with a narcotic, along with an antinausea medication. Newer options may include the use of a one-time injection of the NSAID Toradol (ketorolac) or an intravenous (IV) migraine "cocktail" involving a mix of medications often involving an antihistamine and an antiinflammatory, sometimes combined with a small amount of narcotic.

- Over-the-counter (OTC) migraine preparations such as Excedrin migraine may be effective for some patients but it is important to note that even these medications, if taken frequently, can lead to medication overuse headache. NSAIDs can help to reduce inflammation and may be an effective treatment for a mild to moderate migraine if taken in the early stages. But NSAID medications will not help with other associated symptoms such as nausea, vomiting, or sensory disturbances, and they may worsen gastrointestinal symptoms.

- Aspirin has long been an important OTC treatment for headaches of all types and now a recent study shows that aspirin given IV may be an effective treatment for severe headaches and migraine.

Although not commonly used in the United States, IV-aspirin is "cost-effective, safe, and easy to use...," according to the study's authors, and study participants found the treatment moderately effective about 40% of the time. Aspirin may also be given in a single large oral dose for acute migraine, sometimes with an anti-emetic to reduce symptoms of nausea and vomiting. Potential side effects of aspirin include gastrointestinal distress, bleeding, and rash, and sometimes more serious effects including worsening asthma and kidney damage.

What Nurses Know...

GETTING TO KNOW THE TRIPTANS—
ACUTE TREATMENT FOR MIGRAINE HEADACHES

In the past decade triptans have become the most commonly prescribed medication used to treat migraines. They are usually most effective in halting a migraine when used early in the headache. In addition to relieving headache pain, triptans are also effective in relieving other symptoms associated with migraine, such as nausea, and sensitivity to light and sound. One of the curious things about triptans is that results are highly individualized and you may need to try several different formulations to find the one that works best for you. Triptans work by constricting blood vessels in the brain, relieving swelling caused by inflammatory chemicals, and helping to balance levels of the neurotransmitter serotonin. Triptans appear to have a good safety record but can interact with other medications such as those used to treat depression, including both selective serotonin reuptake inhibitors (SSRIs) and monoamine oxidase inhibitors (MAOIs).

Triptans may also interact with the drug lithium. Because triptans are vasoconstrictors , they should not be used in combination with ergot-derived drugs Dihydroergotamine and ergotamine, or with Sansert (methysergide)—a synthetic ergot-like compound; triptans should not be combined with other types of triptans or any other vasoconstricting medications within a 24-hour period; and triptans should not be used by persons with uncontrolled high blood pressure or in persons with restricted blood flow to the cardiovascular system, the brain, or the extremities. If used with the beta-blocker Inderal (propranolol), Maxalt (rizatriptan) should be used at the lower 5 mg dose. Side effects of triptan medications can include, but are not limited to: dizziness, drowsiness, flushing, mild weakness, and feeling warm or cold. Nasal spray forms can temporarily leave a bitter taste in the back of the throat, and the injectable forms can cause burning at the injection site. Signs of an allergic reaction, which are not common, include a red itchy rash and difficulty breathing. Triptans available on the market at the time of publication include:

- *Amerge—Naratriptan tablet*
- *Axert—Almotriptan—tablet*
- *Frova—frovatriptan—tablet*
- *Imitrex—Sumatriptan—injection, tablet, or nasal spray*
- *Maxalt—Rizatriptan—tablet*
- *Relpax—Eletriptan hydrobromide—tablet*
- *Treximet—Sumatriptan with Naproxen sodium (an NSAID)—tablet*
- *Zomig—Zolmitriptan—tablet or nasal spray*

Prevention

Because those who suffer migraines are extremely sensitive to changes in both internal and external environments, they have a powerful incentive to closely follow the rules of healthy living in order to avoid frequent headaches. For a migraineur almost anything can trigger a migraine: exposure to hormonal fluctuations, stress, dehydration, individual food sensitivities, overexertion, bright reflections or flashes of light, loud, discordant, or irritating sounds, over-stimulation, elevation changes, weather-related barometric pressure changes, excessive heat, and even noxious odors such as cigarette smoke. For some of these reasons, travel can be difficult for those who experience migraines. Overall, for migraine headache prevention, many patients find it is best to avoid disrupting daily routines. Equilibrium: It's a good thing!

A paced program of regular, moderate, aerobic exercise may help to reduce the number of headache attacks in migraineurs as well as increase their overall fitness level—comparable to the effect of the popular migraine-prevention drug (Topamax) topiramate. A Swedish study showed that patients benefitted from 40 minutes of exercise three times per week by experiencing fewer headaches. Other studies showed reductions in headache intensity and the amount of medication used. Further studies may help to refine our knowledge of the most appropriate level and types of exercise for migraine patients, and identify more clearly how exercise leads to improvements in headache status.

If you suffer from migraines, it may be a good idea to review the risk factors and headache triggers in Chapter 2, paying special attention to dietary, environmental, and sensory triggers. If you continue to experience migraine headaches that interfere with your daily life, suffer attacks that last 3 or more days at least twice a month, fail to

What Nurses Know...

Interestingly, there are some commonalities in the way that Western Medicine and Traditional Chinese Medicine (TCM) view causal factors in migraines. Both traditions cite emotional stress, missed meals, physical exhaustion, alcohol, smoking, chocolate, coffee, and dairy products as common triggers. In TCM, the explanations for why these factors contribute to headaches often involves a stagnation of "Qi"—the basic life force or energy, while Western Medicine has other evidence-based explanations.

respond to acute medications, or suffer from headaches more frequently than an average of 2 days per week, a preventative medication is a wise option for reducing headache frequency. A reasonable goal of preventive treatment is to reduce headache frequency and severity by 50%. Patients with less severe headache might see greater success, but becoming entirely headache-free may not be realistic for all people. It may help to remember that migraine is a genetic, neurobiological disorder, and while a complete cessation of headaches might be the Holy Grail, successful headache management that leads to an improved quality of life is an important and realistic goal.

When beginning any new medication for the prevention of migraine, people should be aware that it may take 8 to 12 weeks to determine whether a medication is effective, and more than one medication may need to be trialed.

- Some of the earliest medications used for migraine prevention were the tricyclic antidepressant amitriptyline and the related drug nortriptyline. Other prophylactic medications include the anticonvulsants Topamax (topiramate) and Depakote (divalproex sodium).
- The beta-blocker Inderal (propranolol) is also used successfully in the prevention of migraine and cluster headache. Other beta-blockers used in migraine prevention include atenolol, nadolol, and timolol, as well as the newer medication carvedilol, which seems to have fewer cardiac and cardiovascular side effects.
- Calcium channel blockers such as verapamil help to stabilize blood vessels and reduce vasoconstriction, but it is not clear how they work in migraine prevention, and this is considered an off-label, but common, use. Although there are many different calcium channel blockers, verapamil has the best record of effectiveness in migraine prevention. These medications generally have few serious side effects, but constipation, dizziness, swelling in the legs, and slow or irregular heart rhythm have been reported.
- For about a decade, headache specialists have been treating migraine patients with a formulation of botulinum toxin A, but results have been conflicting. The benefits of Botox were first discovered serendipitously when patients undergoing cosmetic facial treatment with began reporting reduced headache frequency, severity, and duration. The Food and Drug Administration (FDA)

has been studying the efficacy of "Botox" in headache prevention for some years and has not yet approved it for routine migraine treatment. But, in late 2010, Botox was approved for the treatment of chronic migraine. In addition to its well-known neuromuscular effect, Botox appears to have other mechanisms that contribute to reducing headache pain, including inhibiting the release of three important neurotransmitters involved in pain and/or inflammation: CGRP, substance P, and glutamate.

- There are several drugs with newer applications for migraine prophylaxis, including Tizanidine—a short-acting muscle relaxant that inhibits release of the neurotransmitters that cause vasoconstriction and vasodilation; Seroquel (quetiapine)—a short-acting antipsychotic drug that may be useful for patients with headaches resistant to other migraine medications; and Keppra (levetiracetam), an antiseizure drug that may be useful for patients who have migraine with aura.

- Of complementary and alternative medicine (CAM) therapies, acupuncture and craniosacral therapy stand out in their possibilities for treating migraine and are sometimes used together to treat problem headaches. The prodrome or aura periods preceding the headache are thought to be the most effective time to use craniosacral therapy to abort a migraine.

- In two double-blind, placebo-controlled studies, the popular migraine herb "butterbur" proved to be effective in reducing the number of migraine attacks, especially when used at a dose of 75 mg twice daily. Butterbur may be especially useful because of its great tolerability and absence of known drug interactions. There are two important cautions with regard to butterbur:

  1. It cannot be used by pregnant or nursing women.
  2. The preparation used must be a standardized extract that has had the toxic pyrrolizidine alkaloids removed, as they are suspected to cause liver damage.

- Other herbal formulas that stand out include the combination products Migralief (feverfew, magnesium, and riboflavin—vitamin B2), and Migravent (butterbur, feverfew, magnesium, and riboflavin—vitamin B2). Please refer to Chapter 5 for more information.

What Nurses Know...

SEROTONIN SYNDROME

The use of any triptan carries the risk of developing "serotonin syndrome" when used with another triptan or with other medications that increase the availability of serotonin. These include SSRI antidepressants Paxil, Lexapro, and Celexa, MAOIs like Nardil, and tricyclic antidepressants like amitriptyline and nortriptyline. When drugs like triptans are combined with each other or with various antidepressants, excess and prolonged nervous system exposure to serotonin can cause a potentially serious, adverse drug reaction involving: mental confusion, anxiety, and agitation, excessive drowsiness, dizziness, nausea, diarrhea, and autonomic changes indicated by excessive sweating, fever, shivering, and rapid heart rate, high blood pressure, tremors, and seizures. If you develop any of these symptoms while using one of the triptan medications, seek medical help immediately. Symptoms are usually mild but can be quite acute, and rarely, even fatal. Patients taking only triptans or only an SSRI are at very minimal risk but when these two medications are used simultaneously, as is the case with roughly 20% of migraineurs, there is increased concern, because both drugs can increase the amount of circulating serotonin. Overall, the number of patients developing serotonin syndrome annually is quite low, even in patients taking both types of medications—less than 0.03%.

Complications of Migraine

It's well known that a migraine headache can cause temporary neurological symptoms that impair the ability to put thoughts together clearly and can cause other cognitive changes. But can migraine attacks gradually cause accumulated damage to the brain over time? A study using mice as an animal model suggests that the vascular changes associated with migraine closely resemble small "transient ischemic attacks" (TIAs), leaving affected areas of the brain oxygen deficient, and possibly creating permanent changes in the brain.

Dr Takahiro Takano, the study's lead author has said, "In mice, the damage from these episodes looks exactly like the damage that occurs to the brain from repeated TIAs, or transient ischemic attacks," said Takano. "It's long been known that patients having a migraine attack are functionally impaired from the pain. It's also been shown recently that with repeated migraines, a person's cognitive abilities decrease. But actually doing damage to the brain—that is a surprise."

Neuroscientists who work with the brain suggest that migraineurs practice headache prevention by avoiding headache triggers and making use of preventive medications, and that physicians should focus on prevention rather than acute treatment and pain management. So, in the case of migraines, an ounce of prevention really is worth a pound of cure—and if you suffer from frequent migraines, taking a rescue medication alone may not be enough. Speak with your physician about preventive medications or nondrug headache prevention strategies. It's estimated that fewer than 20% of patients who should be taking a preventive medication for migraine currently do so.

A 2011 study suggests that migraine may be a risk factor for cardiovascular disease and stroke, based on findings from a study comparing those with high blood pressure and migraine, versus those with high blood pressure alone. The presence of both hypertension and migraine should prompt physicians to screen for other cardiovascular risk factors at an early age—especially those which are modifiable through medical treatment and lifestyle changes. In the studies done so far, migraine with aura has been most closely associated with increased stroke risk in women. However, it is not clear whether effectively treating migraine can reduce the risk of stroke, and overall, stroke risk is still low.

An Italian study followed over 2,000 patients, of whom 17% had both hypertension and migraine, 43% had hypertension alone, and 40% had migraine alone. This study found that controlling blood pressure proved to be more difficult in patients with both conditions. But the most significant finding was that those who suffered from both hypertension and migraine were up to five times more likely to have suffered a stroke than those with migraine alone. And, in a subgroup of patients aged 40 to 49, the prevalence of stroke or TIA was five-fold greater in the group with migraine and hypertension versus hypertension alone. The majority of patients in the study had migraine without aura, as is also true in the general population.

Variations in Migraine

Migraine is an unusual neurobiological disorder which affects many individuals in different ways. The commonalities include: the tendency for symptoms to be unilateral, or affecting only one side, associated neurological and visual effects, and distinct patterns of onset and resolution. I'll describe several unusual migraine types that can occur often in an individual, or can occur occasionally in a migraineur who also experiences the more common migraine forms.

STATUS MIGRAINOSUS—INTRACTABLE MIGRAINE

When a person has had a continuous migraine headache for more than 3 days, they are said to be in "status migrainosus" (SM). In SM, the headache, most often migraine without aura, is usually severe and debilitating and this sometimes requires hospitalization for IV medications and supportive care. The headache may wax and wane, or even respond temporarily to medications or sleep, but returns relentlessly for periods up to a week or longer. If the headache persists, but the intensity diminishes over time, it may be classified as chronic daily headache, or chronic migraine.

However, the development of migraine-specific medications such as dihydroergotamine and triptans has fortunately limited the number of persistent and intractable migraine headaches. Given the possibility of both damage to the brain and increased risk of stroke, intractable migraine headaches should be treated aggressively from as early as possible in migraine duration.

I unfortunately suffered a period of status migrainousus in the past year. The facial numbness and visual effects associated with my week-long migraine took several additional weeks to resolve completely. It was a very frightening experience that I do not wish to repeat. Now I understand the importance of having a plan in place for a headache that does not respond to my usual treatment methods. Discuss all unusual symptoms following medication changes with your physician, and don't wait—hoping a bad headache will simply subside. Without proper treatment, a severe headache will often persist.

MIGRAINE-ASSOCIATED VERTIGO

I have had long-standing issues with my vestibular system ranging from full-blown vertigo attacks to tinnitus to mild dizziness to distortions in my sense of smell. I've received various diagnoses. The most likely is Meniere's syndrome, but I've not experienced the typical symptoms of Meniere's, which are periodic severe vertigo attacks, with any consistency. These days I would just say I seldom feel tip-top. It's as if my vestibular system is always working overtime.

—D.H.

The cerebellum is the part of the brain that processes information related to movement and balance. Damage to the cerebellum can create problems such as dizziness, nausea, and difficulties with coordination. Dizziness and vertigo are often associated with migraine attacks and both may indicate changes in cerebellar function. Studies show that people who suffer from migraines may have abnormal cerebellar function even *between* attacks, indicated by a lack of fine coordination and differences in visual tracking during movement. The vestibular system, the complex structure in the inner ear made up of a series of circular canals, contributes to our sense of balance and spatial orientation. Abnormalities in the vestibular system have also been found in migraine patients. So, it is not surprising that about half of migraineurs report experiencing motion sickness, far more than those who do not have migraine, and roughly a third of patients experience attacks of vertigo.

We have all experienced dizziness from twirling around too many times as children, from amusement park rides, and from playground equipment. Dizziness feels like we are spinning and cannot keep our balance. Vertigo is a similar, persistent sensation that either we, or our surroundings, are rotating, and this feeling generally becomes worse with movement, especially movement of the head. Vertigo can be accompanied by nausea, vomiting, ringing in the ears, and extreme fatigue and headache. These episodes are different from the momentary light-headedness you may feel after getting up too quickly and they usually last longer—from only a few seconds to many days. Dizziness and vertigo can have many causes, including nervous system and circulatory disorders, drug reactions, food sensitivities, and allergies, but overall, migraine is thought to be one of the most common causes of dizziness and vertigo.

Although not yet recognized by the ICHD-II classification system, *migraine-associated vertigo* (MAV) is a distinct disorder and a common cause of vertigo symptoms, according to specialist Dr Terry Fife. In comparison to people who experience tension headaches, patients with migraines are three times as likely to suffer from vertigo. It's estimated that 3% to 3.5% of Americans have MAV, making it an important cause of episodic dizziness.

Vertigo symptoms can occur before headache onset or during a headache. MAV may also be experienced during a headache-*free* period, with some patients reporting vertigo or dizziness, rather than headache, as the primary symptom. Despite the association between migraine headache and MAV, headache presence is not required to make the diagnosis of MAV. Vertigo may be accompanied by some unusual symptoms including nystagmus—a condition characterized by repetitive uncontrolled rapid eye movement usually affecting both eyes, and often exacerbated by looking in one direction.

There is no specific test for MAV and inner ear tests are usually normal, so diagnosis is based on a thorough workup to eliminate other potential diagnoses. It is helpful to see a doctor who specializes in treating vertigo and/or migraine disorders. If you have MAV, it's important to take precautions to avoid injury from dizziness-related falls and to use whatever means necessary to prevent the episodic migraine-associated attacks that can bring on vertigo. Avoiding common trigger foods and food additives and taking prophylactic medications such as beta-blockers or tricyclic antidepressants are common treatment approaches. Verapamil and amitriptyline are useful because they also have anticholinergic effects that may help control vertigo in addition to their effectiveness in reducing the occurrence of migraine.

MIGRAINE AURA WITHOUT HEADACHE: ACEPHALGIA MIGRAINE

One of the most unusual migraine forms may not include a headache at all. *Migraine aura without headache* is characterized by having at least two visual disturbances or aura-like symptoms, nausea, vomiting, and constipation, but without accompanying head pain or motor weakness. Each attack may last from 5 to 60 minutes and symptoms must be fully reversible. But the defining characteristic is that headache does not occur with the aura or follow within one hour. Headache specialists have suggested that unexplained fever, dizziness, and/or unexplained pain in a particular part of the body could also be possible types of headache-free migraine.

VISUAL SYMPTOMS: RETINAL MIGRAINE AND OPHTHALMOPLEGIC MIGRAINE

In retinal migraine, patients habitually experience attacks of visual disturbances including scintillations (different patterns of twinkling lights), scotoma (localized area of decreased or lost vision), or total or partial temporary blindness—beginning before the onset of migraine headache. For proper diagnosis, these visual effects should be confirmed by examination during an attack, which of course isn't easy to arrange, so physicians may also rely on a patient's careful drawing of their visual field defect—made during the attack. Generally, only one side of the head and one eye are affected. Headache symptoms usually begin within 60 minutes of the first visual symptoms and may last up to 72 hours. They can include a pulsing or throbbing quality and moderate to severe pain which is aggravated by exertion. Nausea (with or without vomiting) and sensitivity to light or sound are usually present. But, two important criteria for diagnosing retinal migraine are that (1) all visual effects must be fully reversible, and that (2) a patient must have a normal ophthalmological examination between attacks. A thorough patient examination and investigation is necessary to rule out other causes of sudden-onset temporary blindness. To meet ICHD-II criteria for retinal headache patients must have experienced at least *two* similar attacks.

Sporadic attacks of retinal migraine are treated with common migraine medications such as NSAIDs, antinausea medications, ergotamines, and triptans. Preventive treatments may be effective for those with frequent attacks. Vision changes in retinal migraine should last only as long as the migraine attack. If vision does not return to normal following the resolution of other symptoms, see your regular doctor or your eye doctor as quickly as possible.

Ophthalmoplegic migraine is a rare occurrence usually linked to vascular changes due to diabetes or carotid artery abnormalities, or to nerve palsy (weakness). Symptoms, which often last for a week or more, include headache, droopy eyelid, dilated pupil, double vision, and weakness or paralysis of the muscles surrounding the eye. In sequence, a migraine-like headache is usually accompanied by or followed within 4 days by eye-related symptoms—caused by pressure on the third, fourth, or sixth cranial nerves. Episodes must occur on *two* separate occasions to meet diagnostic criteria.

Is a Common Heart Defect Related to Migraine?

In the past decade, research has shown that for thousands of people, there is a connection between a common congenital heart defect and migraines with tingling in the extremities and visual aura. Before birth, there is an opening—known as the formen ovale—between the two upper chambers of the heart. This small opening, up to 1 centimeter in diameter, normally closes up immediately after birth, but in as many as a quarter of us it does not close completely—leading to the condition known as patent formen ovale (PFO). (Note: "patent" means "open.") While usually harmless, recent research suggests that migraine with aura is more common in people with PFO and that surgical closure can lead to improvements in migraine symptoms. PFO is also more common in people who have migraine with aura than in the general population but it isn't yet clear whether there is a causal relationship or whether the two disorders coexist for some other reason. We also don't know with certainty why closure of a PFO so often leads to improvement in migraine symptoms. If you suffer from migraine with aura and you would like to be tested for PFO, ask your physician about this possibility.

Could Your Headache be a Migraine?

In summary, migraines are among the most common primary headache types and they're distinguished by a characteristic grouping of symptoms, including those listed below. If your headaches fit this profile, see a doctor for proper diagnosis and treatment.

- Moderate to severe throbbing, pulsating, pain affecting primarily *one* side of the head, often located behind the eye, or in the temple area.
- Sensory disturbances including sensitivity to light and sound, a heightened sense of smell, or an alteration in tactile sensation, such as experiencing pain from usually nonpainful stimuli like brushing the hair or pressing the skin on the back of the head.
- Visual disturbances such as seeing bright lights, experiencing blurry vision (especially at the edges of your field of vision), seeing halos around objects, or seeing wavy lines.
- Dizziness, fatigue, or exhaustion—before, during, or after the headache
- Loss of appetite, nausea, vomiting, or more rarely, abdominal pain (more common in children with headaches).
- Cold hands and/or feet, or other body temperature changes.
- Any of these unusual symptoms occurring before headache onset (during the prodromal or aura phases in migraine).
- Lasting symptoms of unusual weakness, fatigue, foggy thinking, and a feeling of being "wrung out" for up to 24 hours following resolution of the headache.

The next two chapters of the book discuss primary headaches in the context of two special groups, children and teens, and women throughout every stage of life.

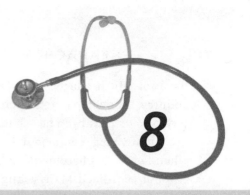

8

Primary Headaches in Children

I felt so bad for my son. Every Monday he would come home from school with a terrible headache, eventually throw up, and fall asleep. No OTC medications seemed to help. Our doctor gave us a list of trigger foods, but avoiding them didn't help either. We finally went to the hospital for a CT scan. Luckily he didn't have a brain tumor. Month after month, he still suffered. We saw a neurologist who offered two different prescriptions that only made my son sleepy. Finally, as a young teen, our family doctor prescribed a very light dose of amitriptyline, and we even cut it in half. That was the only thing that helped, although it didn't take them completely away. Now age of 22, he still gets headaches, but not as often. KIM

Any parent knows that watching a child suffer with chronic headache pain can be heartbreaking. But how common are headaches in children? Very—headaches account for 20% of pediatric outpatient visits to primary care physicians and 57% to 82% of preteens and teenagers have episodic headaches. Incidence of headaches in children varies by country. For example, 39% of children under six in Sweden and 85% of 15-year-olds in Taiwan have had headaches. Before puberty, headaches are slightly more common in boys, but the ratio changes after puberty when headaches become much more common in girls and remain so through adulthood. Many young children seem to suffer from migraine-like attacks that last less than an hour, but if the headaches are frequent, medical consultation should be considered. Tension headaches are also common, especially in adolescents. And, unfortunately, a small number of children also suffer from chronic daily headaches.

Causes and Risk Factors

A large Brazilian study involving over 2,000 children found several important factors in the prevalence of migraine, tension-type headaches (TTH), and chronic daily headaches, including the environmental influences and family history outlined below:

- Children with *prenatal tobacco exposure* were much more likely to experience chronic daily headache. Nicotine affects neurotransmitter receptors in the fetal brain, which may ultimately lead to changes in communication between neurons in the brain.
- The risk of chronic daily headache more than doubled in children born to mothers who used *alcohol* during pregnancy.
- Lifetime family headache history, particularly *maternal headache history*, also had a bearing on both headache prevalence and headache frequency: When mothers experienced chronic daily headache, risk of chronic daily headache in children increased more than 12-fold. Other studies of headache frequency in children also suggest that both the *presence* and *frequency* of headache have a familial tendency.

The Brazilian study also identified other health conditions that were more common both in children with migraine headache and to a lesser extent, TTH, including:

- Motion sickness
- Benign paroxysmal vertigo of childhood

- Teeth grinding
- Sleep walking and sleep talking
- Recurrent abdominal pain

All of these disorders were more common in children with episodic migraine, probable migraine, and chronic daily migraine—than in a control group. They also looked closely at a suspected connection between *attention deficit hyperactivity disorder* (ADHD) and headaches in children and found that diagnosis of ADHD was not closely associated with headache disorders in children. But, they did find that hyperactivity and impulse control symptoms were significantly increased in migraine with or without aura, probable migraine, episodic TTH, and probable TTH. These disorders share difficulties in regulating inhibitory systems in the brain.

Primary Headaches in Children

Migraines and TTHs are the most common primary headache conditions in kids, with migraines being more common in childhood, and tension headaches dominating in adolescents. These two conditions can also present as recurrent episodes, or, if occurring 15 or more days per month for 3 months or more, as chronic daily headache. Parents need to be aware that children often have slightly different headache characteristics than adults, and there are some migraine variants that occur in children that rarely if ever occur in adults (see below).

Headaches have huge educational, social, and recreational impacts on the lives of children. When headaches are frequent or chronic a child's quality of life may be greatly reduced. Parents are affected, too, and many find it quite stressful to care for their children with headaches—and to find them appropriate treatment. It may be reassuring to know that most headaches in children are not indicators of serious health conditions and that they can be successfully managed.

PREPARING FOR THE DOCTOR'S VISIT

Diagnosing and treating childhood headaches can be difficult for doctors for a variety of reasons. Headache symptoms are usually subjective, and children can be less than accurate historians, as they do not have the same communication skills as adults. This presents a special challenge for pediatricians because these same factors make it easy to underestimate and undertreat headaches in children. If you think your child might have trouble describing headache symptoms it may be helpful to suggest that your child to think about this ahead of the doctor's visit. Encourage the use of descriptive terms, and if visual symptoms are present, ask the child to draw a picture of what they see. But there is a fine line between preparing your child for a visit to the doctor and "coaching" a child on what to say. Since headache symptoms are subjective, it is important for the child to relate what was experienced as accurately as possible in order to aid the doctor in making the correct diagnosis and ordering appropriate treatment.

OBTAINING A DIAGNOSIS

At the doctor's office or emergency room a thorough medical history and physical exam is usually all that is needed to diagnose most primary headaches in children. Children with a history of head trauma, stiff neck, and worsened head pain with neck movement, photophobia, fever, decreased level of consciousness or awareness, seizure history, or abnormal neurological exam require more extensive laboratory testing and may require diagnostic imaging such as a high-quality head CT. Children who have a known history of seizure disorder should have blood levels of anticonvulsant medications

What Nurses Know...

Studies show the importance of establishing strict guidelines for use of neuroimaging in children with recurrent headaches: The rate of abnormal findings on neuroimaging was highest among those children with a prior abnormal neurological examination (50%) and lowest among children with recent onset of severe headache (7%) and when demanded by parents and/or physicians (10%).

checked if they have a headache. Children needing further evaluation will usually be referred to an appropriate specialist.

Family history, too, can be valuable in helping to diagnose pediatric headaches. Roughly 70% of children with migraine-like symptoms have a family history of migraine and the condition should be suspected in children with recurrent episodes of severe headaches.

PREVENTING AND MANAGING HEADACHES IN CHILDREN

Some observant parents can recognize situations and patterns of behavior that will lead to a headache in a child and can change activities or environmental conditions as a preventive strategy. For example, limiting too much "screen time" (TV, computer games, movies), keeping children well-hydrated by offering cool drinks, keeping blood sugar stable by offering healthy snacks, insisting on quiet time to allow a child to destress, and providing alternate activities that promote relaxation. It is sometimes helpful for parent to lay down with a very young child, apply a cool cloth to the child's forehead, and sing softly or read a simple book. These lifestyle modifications can be useful in preventing and managing both tension and migraine headaches. Headache-prone children should be encouraged to follow a regular schedule for meals, bedtime, relaxation periods, and healthy exercise. Obesity and sedentary lifestyle are also linked to childhood and adolescent headaches, and physical exercise can improve the quality of life for many children with frequent headaches.

Clinicians, parents, and children should be observant and consider possible dietary and environmental triggers, including cigarette smoke, in primary headaches like TTH and migraine. Children can be taught at an early age to avoid certain foods or situations that trigger headaches.

TREATMENT OF PRIMARY HEADACHES IN CHILDREN

The short-term goals of treatment are to relieve pain, treat nausea, and enable the child to achieve restful sleep. Sleeping, even briefly, often helps alleviate both TTH and migraine headaches in children. Learning to guide your child through relaxation techniques or working with a professional on biofeedback techniques is also helpful. CAM therapies include acupuncture, naturopathy, and psychological

What Nurses Know...

Some common factors that may trigger migraines in children include the following:

- Stress and anxiety related to school, social, or family situations
- Lack of sleep and disruptions to the child's bedtime routine
- Menstruation and the use of birth control pills in girls
- Overexertion, especially accompanied by dehydration
- Extremes of light, glare, or strobe effects
- Strong, unusual, or chemical odors, such as tobacco smoke
- Failing to eat a healthy diet and skipping meals
- Barometric pressure changes or abrupt high altitude travel such as mountain ski trips.
- Food and beverage triggers including nitrates, sulfites, glutamate and monosodium glutamate (MSG), caffeine use or withdrawal, excess salt, and foods high in tyramine (discussed previously). Cheese, nuts, chocolate, and shellfish are also common triggers. The amino acid phenylalanine is also a possible trigger, but is present in many healthy foods, including most proteins, legumes, some nuts, and some seeds. Phenylalanine can constrict blood vessels and can trigger a migraine in many sensitive people, including children. Phenylalanine is also in the artificial sweetener aspartame which is found in diet sodas and it is easily avoided by not drinking these unhealthful beverages.

counseling support. Very young children may do best with the non-drug and preventive treatments discussed above.

Using medications to treat headaches in children is not simply a matter of adapting adult treatment methods. This is important for two reasons: First—many medications used in adult migraine are not safe to use or have not been proven to be safe to use in young children, and second—in the few studies done in children there is a very high placebo success rate, which makes it unclear whether using these medications in very young children is effective. Children do often respond well to over-the-counter (OTC) analgesics like ibuprofen or acetaminophen but these must not be used frequently or they may cause medication-overuse or "rebound" headache. For this reason, older children and teenagers should be discouraged from self-medicating. In addition, antinausea drugs and other medications are sometimes used. But, pediatricians advise against giving children aspirin, especially when the cause of a headache is unknown because of complications with viruses.

What Nurses Know...

Aspirin can lead to the development of "Reye's syndrome," a life-threatening disease that can cause organ and brain damage in children who have a viral infection, which can be accompanied by headache. The Food and Drug Administration (FDA), Centers for Disease Control and Prevention (CDC), and the American Academy of Pediatrics recommend that aspirin and aspirin-containing medications not be given to children under the age of 19, if fever or a fever-causing viral illness is present. The National Reye's Syndrome Foundation goes so far as to recommend salicylate-containing products not be used at all in children and teens because a viral illness may be present before symptoms are recognized as such. Labels should be screened carefully for alternate words for aspirin, including:

- *Salicylates*
- *Acetasalicylate*
- *Acetylsalicylic acid*
- *Salicylic*
- *Salicylamide*
- *Phenyl salicylates*

Recognizing Serious Warning Signs

Although headaches in children can be very concerning to parents, most are not serious. In unusual circumstances, however, headaches might be related to a secondary illness or condition, and it's important to recognize the more serious signs that a child that requires a complete diagnostic workup. For example, headaches can be a sign of lesions, inflammation, or increased pressure within the skull. Seek medical attention for the indicators listed below:

- New or different headache symptoms or an increase in headache frequency. Any new headache or a recent onset headache with no prior similar episode should be discussed with your medical practitioner. These "acute headaches" could possibly be a result of systemic infection, trauma from head injury, or a first migraine episode, and they need to be properly evaluated.
- A headache that develops after a fall or head injury.
- A headache that also includes symptoms such as vomiting, visual changes, fever, neck pain, or stiff neck.
- Headaches that occur frequently, or that occur in conjunction with frequent use of pain medications or OTC analgesics like ibuprofen or acetaminophen. Children, as well as adults, can develop "medication overuse headache" (also called "rebound headache").
- Headaches that are worse in the morning and improve as the day progresses. (In contrast, many other headaches tend to begin or worsen throughout the day.)
- Headaches that are aggravated by sneezing, coughing, or straining, all of which can temporarily increase intracranial pressure.
- Persistent headaches that are confined to the base of the skull (or occipital region).
- Headaches that worsen in frequency or severity, especially over a short period of time.

Parents need to seek medical treatment as soon as possible for *any* of the above conditions. In addition, any child who shows neurological or behavioral changes related to a headache requires emergency treatment. In the event of a serious pathological cause of headache early diagnosis and treatment is critical.

Tension Headache in Children

TTH is the most common headache type in adolescents and it affects more than twice as many girls than boys. These headaches follow patterns similar to adult TTH, with episodic or chronic forms. The prevalence rate most commonly cited is 15% to 20%. Risk factors for TTH in childhood and adolescence include family history, difficulty managing stress, depression, and poor sleep. Poor posture related to slouching, improperly carried school backpacks, and even the head-forward posture common when texting, may play a role. But recent studies have shown the significance of four major risk factors:

- Obesity
- Sedentary lifestyle
- Alcohol
- Tobacco

SYMPTOMS

Many teens complain of a band-like feeling of tension and pain that begins gradually in the afternoon and lasts from less than an hour to 24 hours. TTH can present with a throbbing pain in the forehead, crown of the head, or can wrap around the base of the skull to encompass both sides of the head. The pain of a full-blown TTH may sometimes have a throbbing quality, but these headaches are not accompanied by the neurological and visual effects of migraine.

Adolescents can also suffer from *combined* TTH and migraine headaches. I recently surveyed my college-age son's friends, many of whom I remembered having tension headaches in junior high. All five young men said they had experienced very frequent headaches through junior high, and that they currently do not get headaches. This same pattern was present in other young male family members. I would like to see a study examining TTH in boys entering puberty, when hormones surge, to determine whether there is a hormonal component.

DIAGNOSIS

The most important factor affecting accurate diagnosis is headache history, and so keeping a headache diary is a great idea. Parents may also be asked to provide more in-depth information on headache history and duration for a young child. If the neurological and physical examinations appear to be normal and headache history is consistent with TTH, additional blood tests and diagnostic scans are rarely necessary.

It is not always easy to tell the difference between TTH and migraines even in adults, and children present special challenges. But an overview of pediatric headaches in emergency medicine revealed some signs to be aware of/look for:

- TTH is more likely to occur during stressful circumstances
- In TTH, discomfort involving the neck and the back of the head is prominent and the muscles of the posterior neck may be tight and painful to pressure
- TTH pain is continuous during an episode
- Nausea and vomiting are not usually present with TTH

TREATMENT

Treating TTH in adolescents is similar to treating TTH in adults and employs the use of OTC medications and nondrug therapies. Ensuring that children and adolescents achieve adequate restful sleep is very important but not always an easy task for parents. In this headache type, it is particularly important to provide strategies to help manage stress. Relaxation exercises and biofeedback may be helpful (see Chapter 5).

For teens with persistent or chronic TTH, prophylactic medications may be used, and might include Elavil (amitriptyline hydrochloride), Topamax (Topiramate), or Periactin (cyproheptadine). The use of habit-forming medications is discouraged. Keeping up with school work is also important, as missed school days can affect teens socially and increase stress related to academic performance. Adolescents have plenty of natural energy and getting at least 30 minutes of exercise three times a week may help in keeping headaches at bay. The Cleveland Clinic also suggests: eating regular meals, drinking 6 to 8 glasses of water daily, applying nondrug comfort measures and acute medications at headache onset (don't wait!), and maintaining regular follow-up visits with the child's physician.

I had heard of migraines for years before my first. I reacted to other people's stories as if they did not have anything really significant. Some classmates would occasionally skip school due to these "earthquakes of the brain" and I even used "a migraine" as an excuse to sit in the nurse's office for the afternoon. I now have a deep respect and sympathy for people who have these terrible episodes and sadly this had to come from my own experience.

I was 12 years old and when the migraine hit I couldn't have spelled my own name if you had asked. It was the first time in my life I felt utterly debilitated. The symptoms came on rather quickly, and suddenly, light, noise, or thinking became a painful burden. I buried my head in the softest cushion I could find—the back seat of my mother's Chrysler. I don't know how long I sat there with my eyes slammed shut, fingers jammed in my ears. By the recount of my parents this excruciating episode began happening about an hour-and-a-half before I starting vomiting. My head was heavy and trying to move even an inch was excruciating. Unlike more common headaches which affect the temples or the back of the neck, this headache hurt everywhere. It all made for a traumatic experience with which nothing else compared.

—RILEY

Migraine Headache and Variants in Children

Migraine headache in children is a serious medical problem, affecting roughly 10% of children and 28% of adolescents. It is now recognized by the International Classification of Headache Disorders-II (ICHD-II) as a distinct disorder. Migraine headaches can begin in early childhood, puberty, the late teens, or in early adulthood. Migraines are the most common primary childhood headache, affecting roughly 90% of pediatric patients seen by neurologists for headache treatment. Roughly 60% of children with migraines are male, although this ratio is reversed after puberty, when migraine becomes much more common in girls. The two major classifications of migraine in children are migraine without aura—distinguished by at least five attacks of pulsating moderate-to-severe headache accompanied by nausea, vomiting, and sensitivity to light or sound, and migraine with aura—which must also include at least two attacks accompanied by aura. Aura refers to the visual distortions such as spots, swirling colors, or flickering lights and other sensory disturbances discussed in Chapter 7.

SYMPTOMS

Children with migraine can present with different symptoms than older teens and adults with migraine and symptoms also vary with the type of migraine. Children often have headache pain on both sides of the head and across the forehead beginning in late afternoon, and headaches may be of shorter duration than in adults. Older teens may have more severe, one-sided migraines that begin earlier in the day. An estimated 14% to 30% of children with migraines experience aura, but the majority of children's migraines occur without aura. Migraines in children are often accompanied by nausea, vomiting, sensitivity to light and sound, and for some, abdominal pain. Children with migraines often have had past episodes of motion sickness, dizziness, or vertigo. Prior to a migraine attack, the child's behavior often shows changes such as irritability, fatigue, and voluntarily withdrawing from social or educational activities. Two-thirds of all kids who have migraines have a family history of migraine.

MIGRAINE VARIANTS

There are some unique variations of migraine that occur almost exclusively in children and only rarely in adults. These "variants" often present with transient neurological symptoms that come before or accompany the headache and can be frightening for both children and their parents. These "complicated migraines" include hemiplegic migraine, basilar migraine, confusional migraine, and benign paroxysmal vertigo of childhood.

Hemiplegic migraine, although also occurring in some adults, is more common in children and is characterized by sudden profound weakness or paralysis on one side of the body (hemiplegia). Feelings of paralysis begin to occur just prior to or during a migraine headache and symptoms can last for several days. Vertigo (a spinning sensation), a pricking or stabbing sensation, and difficulty seeing, speaking, or swallowing may also occur just before the onset of headache pain, and then usually diminish. This migraine disorder often runs in families, where it is known as Familial Hemiplegic Migraine (FHM). In people with FHM, inherited genetic mutations may make the brain more sensitive or excitable, most likely by increasing levels of a chemical called glutamate, a powerful excitatory neurotransmitter released by nerve cells in the brain. But, this form of migraine can also occur in individuals without a family history of the disorder, when it is known as Sporadic Hemiplegic Migraine (SHM). People who experience hemiplegic migraine should carry identification and consider wearing a medical-alert bracelet. If an attack leads to an inability to speak or behavioral problems, it may be difficult to ask for help.

I have had migraines since I was a little girl and I will never forget how painful they felt. But I definitely remember my first hemiplegic migraine. All of a sudden I felt my right thumb go completely numb and then slowly it went from one finger to another. Then I felt the inside of my mouth go numb. Then, I started getting scared because I couldn't speak correctly. My vocabulary words were getting mixed up and I wasn't making any sense. My mother brought me to the ER and they identified it as a Hemiplegic Migraine. The funny thing is that I didn't feel any head pain like with my normal migraine.

—EMILY

I had my first hemiplegic migraine when I was in the 7th grade. My left fingers tingled then went numb, then the left side of my tongue went numb—which made it hard to speak clearly— and I got a really bad headache. For several years before this, I had what doctor would describe as an abdominal migraine. I would get sweaty, extremely weak, and have diarrhea. An hour or so later I would be fine. Later, my migraines progressed to include classic migraine to go along with hemiplegic migraine. I guess I am just prone to migraine disorders.

—ALICIA

Basilar-type migraine, sometimes called "Bickerstaff syndrome," is a form of migraine that mainly affects children and adolescents, and most often teenage girls. Attacks may be timed with the menstrual cycle and begin with an aura that can include a wide array of symptoms, including: dizziness, loss of balance, poor muscle coordination, slurred speech, and tinnitus (ringing in the ears). But, this disorder also includes some frightening and potentially dangerous symptoms, including the possibility of confusion, fainting, blurred vision, and partial or total temporary blindness. These symptoms originate from the brainstem and they can affect both halves of the brain simultaneously. Symptoms may last up to an hour and diminish in the wake of more typical throbbing, pulsating headache pain, which, unlike more common forms of migraine, is felt bilaterally in the back of the head. Patients who experience basilar-type migraines often also experience more typical migraine with aura.

Confusional migraine, more common in boys, is characterized by short-lasting attacks of sensory impairment, agitation (or, extreme lethargy), difficulty speaking, and poor memory. Symptoms are usually relieved by sleep.

Benign paroxysmal vertigo of childhood can include recurrent episodes of difficulty in coordination, balance and walking, a spinning sensation (vertigo), and tilting of the head in children under age 5.

These four migraine-related conditions of childhood are unusual and uncommon. I've mentioned them only because they are part of the childhood migraine spectrum and the preventive strategies and symptomatic treatments for these disorders are often based on the same treatments that work for more typical migraine symptoms. If you would like more information about these disorders speak to a specialist in pediatric neurology.

DIAGNOSING MIGRAINE HEADACHE AND VARIANTS IN CHILDREN

The doctor will question both the child and parents about symptoms and evaluate neurological and visual signs carefully, to exclude other serious disorders and to distinguish possible migraine from TTH. Both pediatricians and parents need to remember that children with migraines may complain of pain on both sides of the head, experience headaches lasting only about an hour, and may suffer additional symptoms involving abdominal discomfort. These characteristics are different from those typically found in adult migraines. For more information, check out "Preparing for the Doctor's Visit" and "Obtaining a Diagnosis" at the beginning of this chapter.

TREATING MIGRAINES IN CHILDREN

Before discussing medications for children with migraines, it is important to mention that treating certain migraine disorders with the usual vasoconstricting medications is contraindicated, and even dangerous. Hemiplegic migraine, for example, should not be treated with triptans, because doing so can increase the risk of stroke. The neurological symptoms in these migraines are caused

What Nurses Know...

Another specific diagnostic feature that parents, and doctors, can look for in children with recurrent headaches is "Red Ear Syndrome" (RES), an uncommon condition characterized by sudden reddening of one or both ears, accompanied sometimes by pain, and by a feeling of burning. The ears actually become hot to touch. RES usually affects both ears and occurs most often in boys. Medications used to treat migraine headache have been used on a trial basis to treat RES, and in late 2010, the journal Cephalgia *reported results clearly showing an association between RES and migraine headache. In the study, RES was reported to occur in more than 23% of children with migraine, in contrast to less than 4% of children with other types of headache. In the majority of RES attacks, symptoms developed during the headache phase of migraine and duration of the attack was variable. Children with RES also report having some migraines that do not include this additional symptom.*

by lack of blood flow to specific areas of the brain and they can be further aggravated by using medications like triptans that narrow blood vessels. Caffeine, tobacco, and other substances that cause vasoconstriction should also be avoided. Other medications such as nonsteroidal antiinflammatory drugs (NSAIDs), antinausea drugs, and analgesics can be safely used to treat hemiplegic migraine. Calcium channel blockers may be effective preventive medications.

The effectiveness of triptans in adolescent migraine has not been thoroughly studied. In fact, most triptans have not yet been approved for use in children and adolescents. But, a new study looking at the effect of a combination of sumatriptan and naproxen sodium, marketed as Treximet, shows a good response in this age group and raised no added safety concerns.

The beta-blockers propranolol and the longer acting nadolol are used to treat pediatric migraine, except in patients with asthma or diabetes.

The tricyclic antidepressant Elavil (amitriptyline) may be used in headache prevention in preteens and teenagers. Periactin (cyproheptadine), a medication with antihistamine, anticholinergic, and antiserotonin properties may be used in younger children. Both amitriptyline and cyproheptadine can be sedating and cause weight gain, but these drugs have a long record of safety and clinical success. Anticonvulsants have also been used as a prophylactic treatment and are especially appropriate when a seizure disorder overlaps with migraine.

What Nurses Know...

Throughout the book I've mentioned the benefits of applying ice or cold packs to the affected area, but for some young children, the cold feeling can be hard to tolerate. Offering the child with a headache a popsicle is an ideal way to apply a cold treatment. It may be most effective for migraine if the child holds or rubs the popsicle against the roof of the mouth while the popsicle melts.

Migraine-Related Abdominal Symptoms in Children

Other important migraine-related disorders in children include abdominal migraine (AM) and cyclic vomiting syndrome (CVS), two migraine variants with pronounced gastrointestinal symptoms. It's common to have nausea and/or vomiting in a migraine attack, but these symptoms can occur repeatedly in children who do not always have accompanying headache.

Abdominal migraine (AM) is a unique form of migraine found almost exclusively in children and teens. In 2004, the ICHD-II coded this disorder under the category "Childhood Periodic Syndrome Precursor of Migraine"—because a large number of children who experience AM will go on as adults to experience other more common forms of migraine headache. AM affects up to 4% of children from about age 7 to 12 or older. AM affects girls more than boys by a slight margin. Although this disorder has distinct diagnostic criteria, it can be overlooked in children for several reasons: First, children are not always able to describe their symptoms adequately, which makes pinning down a diagnosis difficult. Second, doctors can spend considerable time ruling out other important causes of abdominal pain in children, delaying diagnosis. It may take a visit to a neurologist—who might be familiar with the disorder—to identify AM.

SYMPTOMS

Children with this disorder usually experience a sudden onset of intense pain localized in the central abdomen around the navel. Abdominal pain may be accompanied by lack of appetite, nausea, and vomiting. Similarities with migraine include sensitivity to light and a family history of migraine, but headache is present in only a small number of kids. A child may appear pale or flushed and may clutch the abdomen. Although the peak incidence of AM is in 10- to 12 year-olds, it persists into the late teens in more than a third of patients; it rarely persists into adulthood but it is common for symptoms to transform into a more common form of migraine with more typical headache symptoms. AM is episodic, lasting for several hours up to 3 or 4 days, but with no lingering abdominal symptoms following the attacks.

Scientists know there is a close connection between the gut and the central nervous system and most of us realize that stressful situations can have a direct impact on our abdominal functions. Researchers have suggested that in AM, stress-induced release of neurotransmitters and other chemical substances from the central nervous system leads to difficulty in regulating the gastrointestinal system. It isn't difficult to understand how this could lead to nausea and vomiting, but it is more difficult to find a clear explanation for the acute abdominal pain common in AM.

DIAGNOSIS

Few parents would think to approach a neurologist when a child experiences gastrointestinal symptoms, so a pediatrician, pediatric-nurse-practitioner, or even a pediatric gastroenterologist often sees a child initially. It is certainly appropriate to rule out more common causes of episodic abdominal pain and a thorough history and physical is the first place to start. It's helpful for parents to keep an accurate account of the attacks in a symptom diary, including frequency, pattern, duration of pain period, and recurrence. It is also important to note possible precipitating factors—including stress, and to note the success of any attempted treatments such as lifestyle changes. If a child begins to vomit, it is very important to note the frequency and the amount of fluid lost. Children can vomit many times per day and *dehydration is a significant concern.* AM may initially appear to mimic appendicitis or intestinal obstruction, so the physician may order diagnostic imaging. Although noninvasive, these scans can be scary for a young child. Parents and medical staff can help by explaining what to expect in terms the child can understand (see Chapter 4).

AM diagnostic criteria added to the ICHD-II in 2004 require five repeated similar episodes of abdominal pain without other organic cause. This differs from the Pediatric Criteria for Functional Gastrointestinal Disorders (FGIDS), adopted in 2006, which suggests only two such episodes to meet the criteria for AM. Even though headache is not typical of the disorder, when headache does accompany the characteristic symptoms, it helps in making the diagnosis of AM.

In AM, the key feature to look for is recurrent, episodic, intense abdominal pain surrounding the navel, not chronic abdominal pain, and not sudden severe abdominal pain that doesn't go away. There must be distinct symptom-free periods between episodes to fit the diagnosis. According to one study, there are few other reasons for recurrent abdominal pain of this type in young children, and the presumptive diagnosis should be AM, especially if there is a family history of migraine in a parent, older sibling, or grandparent. A long-term study tracking 54 children with AM into young adulthood found that 70% went on to develop migraines as adults.

TREATMENT

The foundation of treatment for AM is strong family education and support—an important nursing role that includes explaining the condition and offering reassurance to worried parents and young patients, careful interviewing to screen for possible environmental, social, or dietary triggers, and coaching families in behavioral therapies. Prevention is also a key in managing AM. Below is a list of possible strategies adapted from an article entitled *Recognizing and Diagnosing Abdominal Migraine* published in the *Journal of Pediatric Health Care*:

- Effective coping strategies to prevent and relieve stress
- Bedtime fiber snack to help avoid hypoglycemia and related acute morning attacks
- Frequent travel stops to prevent motion sickness
- Consistent bedtime routine to prevent altered sleep patterns
- Hat or sunglasses to eliminate glare and diminish bright lights
- A diet low in amines, identified with the letter "C"—chocolate, cocoa, citrus, caffeinated drinks, cheese, and [food] colorings; Also avoid MSG, sulfites, and other food additives
- Consider an elimination diet to identify, and then avoid, specific trigger foods

The goal of treating with medications is to quickly resolve the acute abdominal pain, nausea, vomiting, and other symptoms that have caused the interruption in the child's routine. Options range from preventive medications like low-dose amitriptyline, to treating with safe doses of analgesics well-studied in children, including ibuprofen and acetaminophen. Periactin (cyproheptadine) at a low starting dose at bedtime may be an effective and safe strategy for normal-weight children under age 10.

The FDA has not approved all triptans for use with children and adolescents and a recent literature review found that oral triptans were not beneficial in children with AM. But a 2007 study noted the safety and efficacy of zolmitriptan (Zomig) in nasal spray form, in adolescents. From a practical standpoint, a child who is vomiting repeatedly may be unable to keep an oral medication down long enough for it to work, so a nasal spray is very useful.

Cyclic Vomiting Syndrome

Cyclic Vomiting Syndrome (CVS) is a second migraine-related disorder with gastrointestinal symptoms found in children and it is also thought to be a precursor to adult migraine. A unique characteristic of CVS is its cyclical nature. Attacks tend to reoccur on a very regular, even predictable, basis—often striking at nearly the same time of day, lasting the same length of time, and having the same pattern of symptoms as previous attacks. CVS is relatively common, affecting 2% to 3% of school-aged children.

SYMPTOMS

Children with CVS suffer from episodes of extreme nausea and vomiting continuing for many hours up to several days. As one might imagine this disorder is very concerning to parents, and due to persistent

What Nurses Know...

Long bouts of vomiting may require hospitalization for rehydration with IV fluids. Parents need to reassure children with AM that they will be all right and that they will recover. The severe pain may make some children worry unnecessarily about their long-term health.

vomiting, the risk of children becoming dehydrated is very high. The period between attacks is usually completely normal with no lingering abdominal pain or nausea.

Like adult migraine, CVS has four distinct phases.

1. The symptom-free period between attacks.
2. The prodromal or warning phase that an episode will occur soon: Symptoms typically begin with mild nausea, and for some patients, mild stomach pain.
3. The acute phase, involving extreme nausea, protracted vomiting, inability to keep food and fluids down, pale, ill appearance, serious risk of dehydration, and exhaustion.
4. The recovery phase, beginning with a lessening of nausea and vomiting, the child's color returning to normal, and a feeling of returning to normal health.

DIAGNOSIS

CVS can still be a difficult disorder to diagnose, and it may not be until there is a noticeable, predictable, pattern of reoccurring attacks that the diagnosis of CVS is considered. Many parents, too, are unfamiliar with CVS. For the physician, it may be difficult to distinguish between AM and CVS. Some key differences are:

- In CVS nausea and vomiting are the primary concerns. Pain is secondary and may be mild. In AM pain is more likely to be moderate-to-severe and centered around the navel.
- In CVS symptom duration is more variable, lasting from an hour or two up to four or five days. In AM, symptoms last at least several hours and up to 72 hours without treatment.
- In CVS vomiting is key and must occur at least four times in one hour to meet the diagnosis of CVS. There is no such requirement for AM.

Like migraine, CVS may be triggered by eating certain foods or being exposed to environmental triggers which elicit an inflammatory reaction and nervous system excitation. It is even possible that an infection or virus may be involved in this disorder. It isn't yet known what mechanisms may connect CVS and adult migraine, but it is known that there is a high prevalence of migraine among family members of children with CVS. Children with CVS, their mothers, and grandmothers may have twice the risk of having adult migraine as the general population.

TREATMENT

Parents of children with CVS also need to be supportive, reassuring, and accepting in caring for a child with severe nausea and vomiting. But CVS carries the additional risk of dehydration and parents may need to seek medical attention for treatment with intravenous (IV) fluids. Doctors and nurses need to be proactive in educating parents about caring for a very sick child, learning to recognize signs of dehydration, and recognizing when it is time to seek medical care.

Prevention is *key* in CVS and strategies can include identifying and reducing/avoiding exposure to triggers through diet and lifestyle choices. Parents must also be prepared to treat an attack at its onset with prescription medications when necessary. CVS responds to the same group of medications used to treat migraine, including Inderal (a beta-blocker), Periactin (an antihistaminic/anticholinergic), and the triptans (serotonin agonists), but the tricyclic antidepressant Elavil (amitriptyline) is the most widely prescribed preventive medication used for CVS. Efficacy rates for Elavil in CVS range from about 52% to 73%, and it is considered the first line of treatment for children over the age of 5.

CAM treatments include taking the supplement Coenzyme Q10, an antioxidant important in cellular energy-metabolism and in immune system function. It is made by the body and may be obtained from dietary sources, including salmon, tuna, liver and whole grains, or taken as a gel capsule or an oral spray. COQ10 has been used in adults in the prevention of migraine headache and some neurological disorders but its safety in children is not well established. However, the use of CoQ10 in the treatment of CVS has become popular, which has led to recent studies demonstrating its effectiveness. When twenty-two patients taking CoQ10 were compared against patients taking amitriptyline, both groups reported similar reductions in nausea and vomiting, and in frequency and duration of attacks. But CoQ10 had the welcome advantage of having virtually no side effects, while 50% of patients taking amitriptyline reported side effects, severe enough to result in 21% of patients stopping treatment. Other benefits of CoQ10 included greater satisfaction and lower out-of-pocket cost. Additional studies found the amino acid L-carnitine and vitamin B2 (riboflavin) to be helpful in prevention of CVS and migraine related disorders. Be sure to discuss all medications, supplements, herbs, and CAM treatments with your physician before treating your child. For more information on CVS see the Cyclic Vomiting Syndrome Association website: www.cvsaonline.org.

Migraine disorders in childhood can be a serious problem. Occasionally, migraines cease during childhood, perhaps to reappear later in life, while for other children migraines continue to be a life-long struggle.

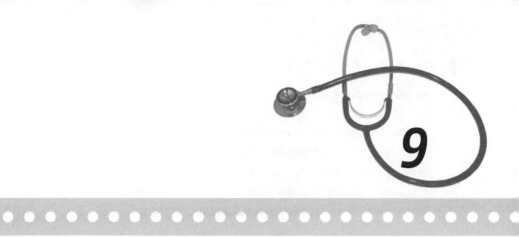

Headaches in Women Through the Lifespan

I often had migraine headaches a day or two before my period started, leaving me unable to do anything for up to two days. But I began to notice that I would not have a headache if I took very good care of myself during the week before my period: I could not skip meals and I had to get a full night's sleep. Most importantly, I had to avoid getting overheated or dehydrated during this critical time. These factors were difficult to manage if I had any project that required my full attention. I am an artist, and the energy required to get a show completed often left me vulnerable to a headache. I once had an art opening that left me so sick I went directly home afterward and threw up.

I thought that my migraines might be related to estrogen levels: When I was on the pill I would always get a headache about forty-eight hours after I stopped taking the hormone part of my Microgestin pack. I talked to my gynecologist about taking the hormone part every day and she agreed I should try it. Previously, I had been taking several different migraine medicines without success—none of them helped much and one of them turned my fingers numb for hours. Taking the hormone part of my pill everyday made a huge difference! I no longer experience a monthly migraine, so I can make plans for any day of the month. I still get an occasional tension headache if I am stressed or I don't take care of myself properly, but the intensity and duration are much less severe than those dreaded pre-menstrual migraines. JULIE

As you have learned in previous chapters, women get more headaches than men during most of the lifespan, especially from puberty through menopause. Prior to puberty, there is not as much difference in prevalence of migraine between genders. During the female reproductive years, migraines are about three times as common in women as in men, mostly because of the increased prevalence of migraine without aura. Why are there such differences in headaches between genders? An important reason is that the sex hormones estrogen and progesterone, which help to regulate menstrual cycles and maintain healthy pregnancies, may affect chemicals in the brain that play a role in the development of many headaches in women. Headache patterns can vary tremendously in times of significant hormonal shifts, including: while taking hormone-stabilizing birth control pills, during pregnancy, immediately after delivery and during the extended postpartum period, and after the roller-coaster of menopause has passed.

Managing headaches adds to the burden of women's lives and makes it even more difficult to juggle career, social activities, and family life. I'll provide a brief overview of headaches during these important stages of life, explore the reasons for headaches in women, and discuss some possible ways to reduce their frequency and severity.

Menstrual Migraine

Many women first begin to experience headaches in their teens with the onset of puberty and monthly menstruation. In fact, headache is a common symptom of premenstrual syndrome (PMS). Approximately, 60% of women who experience migraine without aura associate at least some of their migraine attacks with monthly menstrual cycles. Research beginning in the 1970s suggests that female hormones, especially estrogen, are important factors primarily in migraine without aura in women, perhaps in combination with the effects of inflammatory prostaglandins (hormone-like molecules that act as chemical messengers in the inflammatory response). The total drop in estrogen, from peak to trough, is greater in women with menstrual-related migraine than in women who do not experience these cyclical headaches. And it's thought that this fall in serum estrogen, preceded by several days of peak levels of estrogen, may trigger menstrual migraine. This is known as the "estrogen withdrawal theory," and it helps to explain why women often experience migraine during the placebo week of oral contraceptives, as illustrated by Julie's story at the beginning of this chapter.

Another problem that may contribute to migraines in women is estrogen dominance—having too much estrogen relative to progesterone. Progesterone "opposes" or helps to balance the effects of estrogen. In women with estrogen dominance and migraine, regular use of natural progesterone cream may help reduce headaches; but if headaches are unrelated to hormonal fluctuations, or women do not have estrogen dominance, adding progesterone is less likely to help. A combination of these factors may play a role in women with hormonally influenced headaches like menstrual migraine. Decreasing estrogen levels can trigger headaches or make them worse, but estrogen levels that are too high can also trigger headaches. Equilibrium—it's a good thing!

SYMPTOMS

Symptoms are virtually the same as migraine without aura—moderate to severe one-sided headache with sensitivity to light or sound, nausea or vomiting, and possibly, neurological symptoms that precede or occur during the headache—but menstrual migraine may also be associated with premenstrual symptoms including weight changes, bloating, fatigue, and irritability.

DIAGNOSIS

Pure menstrual migraine is defined as migraine without aura that occurs exclusively within a period spanning from 2 days before to 2 days after the first day of menstruation, in at least two out of three menstrual cycles. These pure menstrual migraines, which affect only about 10% of women with menstrual-related headaches, occur only when estrogen levels begin dropping precipitously and at no other time in the month. Menstrual-related migraines also tend to occur when menstruation begins, but attacks of migraine without aura during the nonmenstrual period may also occur. As defined by the International Classification of Headache Disorders-II (ICHD-II), these menstrual-associated headaches do not involve aura. "Pure menstrual migraine without aura" and "menstrual-related migraine without aura" may be subtypes of migraine without aura, but at least one recent study suggests that menstrual-associated migraine attacks are more intense and longer-lasting than other forms of migraine without aura. You may find, as I have, that menstrual migraines are more persistent and less responsive to your usual migraine medications. An accurate diary tracking menstrual cycles and headaches for a minimum of three months is necessary in order to diagnose menstrual-related migraine.

TREATMENT

Migraines that are known to occur in a cyclical pattern can be treated with the same symptomatic medications used in acute migraine, including triptans like Imitrex and Maxalt, or even by taking OTC medications (see Chapter 7). Nondrug treatments can include the application of an ice-pack or gently massaging the back of the neck and over the entire scalp. Because menstrual-related migraines are cyclical and pure menstrual migraines are predictable, treatments should also include a strong focus on prevention. For women who experience three or more severe headaches a month a prophylactic medication is useful and is usually most effective when taken beginning several days before menses and continuing through the first few days. Women with irregular periods may benefit from a daily preventive medication.

Birth control pills, or oral contraceptives, can have powerful effects on headaches in women. For some women, beginning birth control pills for the first time can trigger the initial onset of new headaches like migraines. Other women experience a variety of changes to different contraceptives, with some worsening headaches and some providing relief. It may also take the body some time to adapt to changes in hormone levels, so although beginning a new birth-control pill may temporarily induce headaches, they may later taper off. It's important to communicate with your doctor if you begin experiencing headaches while on birth control pills because simply adjusting doses or changing the type of pill you are taking may help to alleviate your headaches.

Women who experience migraines and take oral contraceptives are also more likely to suffer a migraine on the days when they take placebo pills. The Mayo clinic has suggested eliminating the placebo days to keep estrogen levels more stable, using an estrogen-releasing skin patch during the placebo week, or switching to a progestin-only pill. Another alternative is switching to a low-dose birth control pill that follows a 24/4 formula containing four placebo pills per cycle rather than the usual seven (21/7 formula), and that also contains the progestin "drospirenone." A recent 60-patient study from Italy on women with pure menstrual migraine showed that groups taking either the 21/7 or 24/4 formula birth control pills were able to reduce their pain level, but those taking the 24/4 formula experienced greater reductions in pain as well as a modest decrease in headache frequency. Both Julie's story, at the beginning of the chapter, and Louise's story, below, illustrate the effect of oral contraceptives on headaches perfectly:

My worst headaches do not fit the description for classic migraines but they are just as disabling. My first one, at the age of 36, came after the birth of my second child. I had started a new birth control pill and when I went on the placebo week of my pills, I got one of these "hormonal" headaches. I remember driving with my two girls and having to pull over to the side of the road to call a friend. My head hurt terribly, I was nauseated, I didn't feel safe driving the car, and I needed help. The symptoms could be likened to the worst hangover of your life. My friend came to pick us up, dropped me off at home, and took care of my kids. I took Extra-Strength Tylenol, went to bed in the fetal position, and awoke about two hours later feeling normal. It wasn't until it happened again two months later during the placebo week of my birth control pack that I made the connection. I am now on a different pill and I rarely get such bad headaches. If I feel one coming on, whether caused by hormonal changes or stress, I try to take an OTC pain reliever (acetaminophen or ibuprofen) before

it gets out of hand, and I continue the medication until the pain is
knocked out or I can go to bed and sleep it off.

—LOUISE

However, it must be noted that as reported in the *British Medical Journal*, a Danish study released in 2011 found that some newer forms of progesterone in combination birth control pills carry an increased risk of blood clots, including pulmonary embolism and those that travel through the circulatory system to cause strokes. Older formulations of oral contraceptives also carry increased risk for developing blood clots, but the risk appears to be roughly half that associated with the newer oral contraceptives. Compared to women not taking any oral contraceptives, those taking a formulation containing both a form of estrogen plus drospirinone face an increased risk of venous thromboembolic events of 6.4%. The absolute risk remains small, at about 10 in 10,000, but multiplied by the number of women taking these products, it is a significant consideration, and must be taken into account in your overall treatment plan.

PREVENTION AND NONDRUG APPROACHES

Balancing and stabilizing hormones may help, and the methods of doing so range from hormone replacement therapy to taking herbal supplements (such as black cohosh) as recommended by a qualified herbalist, or a naturopath specializing in botanical medicine. I also recommend focusing on improving overall health by making use of many of the preventive strategies mentioned throughout the book:

- Keep blood sugar stable
- Eat a balanced, plant-focused whole foods diet
- Drink adequate water
- Avoid the dehydrating effects of caffeine and alcohol
- Stay regular with natural fiber
- Take supplemental magnesium and supplemental vitamin B6 and B2
- Take probiotics to maintain healthy digestion

Women may find it helpful to avoid typical migraine trigger foods, food additives, and processed sugary foods, and to consume ample amounts of antiinflammatory Omega-3 oils.

Exercise is also extremely important at every stage of women's lives, helping them build strong bones in younger years, maintain fitness during pregnancy, age gracefully, and preserve joint flexibility, strength, and balance in later years. But one of the key benefits of exercise is its role in stress reduction. Exercising regularly really can help to reduce the frequency of headaches, as many studies support. Practices that focus on posture, proper breathing, and stretching may be particularly helpful. Consider taking a yoga, Pilates, tai chi, or chi gong class from an experienced instructor. Classes exist at all levels.

Headaches during Pregnancy and the Postpartum Period

As we learned with menstrual migraine, there is a relationship between migraine headaches and changes in estrogen levels. In pregnancy, estrogen production gradually increases to a high point which is then sustained for many months, without the monthly fluctuations that occur during a normal menstrual cycle. As a result, many women experience a welcome decrease in migraine frequency for much of their pregnancy, especially in the calm middle trimester, and for some, migraines disappear completely. Even in the minority of migraineurs who experience an increase in headaches in the first trimester during the ramp-up in estrogen, the remainder of pregnancy usually brings about a significant decrease in headaches.

MILD HEADACHES IN PREGNANCY

Although severe headaches in pregnancy are uncommon and sometimes a cause for concern, experiencing other, less serious, headaches is not an uncommon complaint in women during the first trimester— a time when hormones surge and the volume of blood circulating throughout the body increases. Pregnancy is also a time when women stop using caffeine—which can trigger withdrawal headaches. Some of the factors discussed in Chapter 2, such as sleeping difficulties, low blood sugar, dehydration, poor posture, and stress can also continue to contribute to headaches during pregnancy. What most people refer to as an "ordinary" or common headache is a tension-type headache (TTH) and the usual over-the-counter (OTC) treatments like aspirin and ibuprofen aren't recommended in pregnancy. But for most women, properly dosed acetaminophen is safe for use during pregnancy. All patients must be sure to check with their health practitioner before taking any medications. Overall, the best "treatment" for headaches in pregnancy is prevention.

PREVENTING HEADACHES IN PREGNANCY

If you do occasionally get a tension headache, lying down quietly for a while, practicing deep breathing and relaxation, or applying a flexible cold pack to your head or the back of your neck may be enough to help relieve your discomfort. A warm compress across the bridge of the nose and covering both eyes can sometimes help ease the pain and pressure of sinus headaches. In general, the nasal cavities are more sensitive in pregnancy; inhaling steam during a hot shower or by leaning over a basin filled with hot water with the head covered by a thick towel can sometimes provide relief. A massage focusing on your head, neck, and shoulders or alternating heat and cold applications both help to stimulate blood circulation and can be effective pain-relieving strategies. In addition to massage, acupuncture and biofeedback are other CAM therapies that may be useful for preventing and treating pregnancy-related headaches (see Chapter 5). Vitamin B6, or pyroxidine, may help reduce headache frequency and nausea with migraine. (In some cases, physicians may use Emetrol to control nausea, and if necessary, prescription antinausea medications.) The use of topical remedies like essential oils of lavender and peppermint, in the form of a "Migrastick" or other brand, is controversial in pregnancy, so discuss this with your physician. Below are some additional suggestions:

- Taking a prenatal yoga class or working with a physical therapist may help you maintain proper posture, especially important during the last trimester of pregnancy when the growing weight of your abdomen pulls on the muscles of your lower back and extends muscle tension up the spine to the head and neck.
- Make a conscious effort to avoid stress, go to bed early, and get plenty of sleep. Taking an afternoon nap is helpful to many women, and if possible, it is a good practice to extend into the baby's first months of life, as you learn to "sleep when the baby sleeps."

- It is also healthful and stress-relieving to include moderate exercise. Doing so may help you to avoid several other problems women complain of during pregnancy, such as constipation and hemorrhoids, and it may help you to avoid headaches as well.
- Focusing on nutrition and eating healthy, well-balanced meals is important for you and your growing baby, and it may help prevent headaches. Try to keep your blood sugar stable and decrease gastrointestinal discomfort in later pregnancy by eating five or six smaller meals more spaced throughout the day, rather than three large meals.
- It may be important for you to avoid common food triggers like chocolate and other forms of caffeine, alcohol, foods high in tyramine such as aged cheeses and preserved meats, peanuts, and wheat. Keeping a headache diary can help you to pinpoint which foods are problematic for you. But, it is especially important to avoid overly restrictive diets during pregnancy and breast-feeding.

If you're a migraineur, or you begin to suffer headaches in pregnancy, the most important things you can do are to keep your health care practitioner informed, follow rules for safe medication use during pregnancy, and learn to recognize important warning signs so that you and your doctor can take immediate appropriate action. Headaches during the third trimester are especially concerning, as they may be caused by a condition called "preeclampsia," which can result in dangerously high blood pressure during pregnancy, during childbirth, and in the immediate postpartum period.

Cardiovascular risk, including the risk of heart disease, thrombosis (the development of blood clots in the veins), and high blood pressure, is increased during pregnancy due to the additional circulatory burden. In particular, women with migraine headaches during pregnancy face a 15-fold increase in risk of stroke, although the overall risk of stroke is still low, about four cases in 100,000 births. British researchers, who conducted an analysis of nearly 34,000 pregnancies, concluded that health care practitioners should pay "special attention" to pregnant women with migraines, and to use the opportunity to evaluate the risk of cardiovascular problems. This could also include educating patients about other, modifiable cardiovascular risk factors such as smoking, inactivity, obesity, and poor diet.

What Nurses Know...

WARNING SIGNS IN PREGNANCY

Always speak with your health care provider before taking any new medications, and if the medications you are taking do not relieve your headaches. Let your doctor know immediately if you have any of the following:

- *Headaches that worsen or persist despite appropriate treatment.*
- *Headaches different from those you're used to experiencing, or a new headache in pregnancy; your doctor will want to question you to determine whether the problem could be serious.*
- *A sudden explosive headache so severe that it awakens you from sleep.*
- *Headaches accompanied by blurry vision, swelling in the hands, face, ankles, and feet, especially if accompanied by sudden weight gain, rising blood pressure, nausea, vomiting, fluid retention, or pain in the upper right abdomen. These could be signs of preeclampsia—a potentially life-threatening condition for both mom and baby.*
- *Any headache accompanied by changes in behavior or alertness, fever, stiff neck, drowsiness, slurred speech, or sensation (such as numbness, tingling, or weakness in the face, arm, or leg).*
- *A headache that occurs after a fall.*
- *A persistent headache accompanied by sinus congestion, pain in the forehead or beneath the eyes.*

MANAGEMENT OF PROBLEM HEADACHES DURING PREGNANCY

Although about 85% of women notice a significant reduction in headaches by the second semester, not all women are so fortunate.

Interestingly, women with migraine tend to fare slightly better than women with TTH. Women continuing to have headaches after the first trimester, when things tend to settle down, should discuss both traditional and alternative treatment options with their doctors. I've discussed some possible solutions below.

An article written by headache specialist physician Dawn Marcus for the ACHE Newsletter helps explain why not all women with headaches see a decrease in frequency with pregnancy:

> *"Headache symptoms occur as the result of changes in the brain and nervous system, muscles and joints, blood vessel tone, and psychological variables. Although changes in estrogen reduce activity of pain-activating nerve messengers with pregnancy, estrogen also influences other organ systems with resultant increase in headache susceptibility. Under the influence of high estrogen, blood vessels are more susceptible to constriction and joints are more flexible and lax, both conditions that increase risk of headache…"*

There are other variables that may contribute to headaches in pregnant women, including those with preexisting headache conditions and some women who did not previously experience frequent headaches—including: stress-inducing social and lifestyle changes, fatigue, sleep problems, mood instability, and a tendency to retain fluids. Individual women may respond to these factors in a way that aggravates or triggers chronic headaches. A number of women don't adjust well to stopping the preventive medications they were taking before becoming pregnant.

DIAGNOSTIC HEADACHE WORKUP WHILE PREGNANT

If you do experience a severe, potentially dangerous headache while pregnant, the American College of Radiology recommends MRI without contrast to avoid exposure to ionizing radiation. Studies of toddlers exposed to MRI testing during pregnancy and the offspring of female MRI technicians have not identified significant health problems.

TREATMENT OPTIONS FOR PROBLEM
HEADACHES DURING PREGNANCY

First, it is important to consider all of the preventive strategies mentioned previously, including non-drug treatments like biofeedback and stress management and lifestyle changes like getting more fresh air and moderate exercise. Even if you do end up using medications, these safe strategies will increase your chances of effective headache management.

The use of triptans in pregnancy is controversial, mostly because there isn't yet enough evidence to make a general statement that all triptans are safe. Sumatriptan, which has been around the longest, has also been the best-studied and so far the evidence is reassuring. Although there is not much data suggesting that the use of triptans could lead to birth defects or early miscarriage, there may be data to suggest a link between triptans and premature birth, as well

What Nurses Know...

Although many women would like to avoid using any medications during pregnancy, surveys show that up to one-third of women do, especially to help with pain. Acetaminophen, as mentioned previously, short-acting opioids, and some antinausea medications may be safe if used only sporadically, but to repeat, all nonsteroidal antiinflammatory drugs (NSAIDs), like ibuprofen, naproxen, and aspirin, should be avoided. None of these medications should ever be used frequently in order to reduce the risk of medication overuse headache (rebound headache). But in early pregnancy, NSAIDs may delay implantation of the fertilized egg in the uterine wall and also may increase the risk of miscarriage. In later pregnancy, NSAIDs have been shown to slow the development of the fetal heart. This is one reason why it is so important to discuss the use of all medications with your physician, especially before and during pregnancy.

as maternal blood loss during labor. Triptans are currently desig-nated "Pregnancy Class C," meaning there isn't yet enough data to determine the absolute safety of the medication during pregnancy. Risks of use must be weighed against possible benefits, in a discus-sion between patients with frequent, severe headaches in pregnancy and their physicians. Safety of triptans during breastfeeding is also undetermined, although preliminary evidence shows there is mini-mal risk.

The good news is that there is a long safety record of using beta-blockers such as propranolol in pregnancy because this drug has been widely used for both headache prevention and to manage high blood pressure, without evidence of harm. The use of medications such as antidepressants and Neurontin (gabapentin) may be considered by some obstetricians.

WARNINGS FOR MIGRAINE PROPHYLAXIS AND TREATMENT IN PREGNANCY: TOPAMAX AND DEPAKOTE

In a very small number of women who experience migraine headaches, frequency of attacks will not decrease or may even increase with preg-nancy. If you are already under a physician's care for migraines and you become pregnant, it is extremely important to contact your doctor immediately! Several anticonvulsant medications also used to prevent migraine can cause birth defects. The Food and Drug Administration (FDA) has issued warnings about two in particular: Topamax and Depakote. According to the FDA alert, Topamax use in pregnancy has been conclusively linked to an increase in cleft lip and cleft palate. Cleft lip and cleft palate are oral-facial defects that can cause prob-lems with nursing, eating, speaking clearly, and sometimes also den-tal and hearing problems. The North American Antiepileptic Drug Pregnancy Registry states the risk of birth defects from Topamax is four times greater than that of other medications used to treat epi-lepsy. The journal *Neurology* in 2008 reported that the risk of cleft palate or cleft lip in infants born to mother's taking Topamax was 11 times higher than that in infants born to women who were not tak-ing medication for epilepsy.

Divalproex sodium is marketed as Depakote, Depakote CP, and Depakote ER. Valproate sodium is marketed as Depacon. Valproic

acid is marketed as Depakene and as Stavzor. All of these medications have been used to prevent seizures in epilepsy and some have
also been used for the prevention of migraine. But reliable research
has shown that the use of these drugs may be harmful to fetal development, and they have been specifically linked to neural tube defects
such as spina bifida. Neural tube defects in babies exposed to these
medications during the first three months of gestation occur with up
to 80 times greater frequency than in the general US population. This
means that in the United States, the risk of neural tube defects in
babies increases from one in 1,500 babies in the general population,
to 1 in 20 babies born to mothers taking Depakote during the first
trimester!

Babies born to women taking Depakote also have an increased risk
of being born with major craniofacial defects, cardiovascular malformations, and malformations involving other body systems. Health
care providers have been urged to discuss these risks with women
who are planning to become pregnant or who *could* become pregnant.
They should also discuss stopping the use of Depakote before and
during pregnancy and using alternative medications and therapies,
especially when used for migraine headache—which is ordinarily not
considered life-threatening. Women taking Depakote who do become
pregnant should contact their physician immediately.

Depakote, Topamax, and related medications should not be stopped
abruptly, even in pregnant women—serious problems can occur.
Patients need to follow physicians' advice about discontinuing certain medications, and about alternative treatments that are safe for
to use. Accordingly, women at risk for becoming pregnant should not
use Depakote or Topamax until they have had a thorough evaluation by
a physician, weighed the risks and benefits, and discussed safer alternatives. If it is agreed that using these medications is the best option,
women of childbearing age (females who have reached puberty and
have not yet gone through surgical or natural menopause) are encouraged to use very strict birth control in order to prevent the potential
occurrence of pain, suffering, and life-long disability in children
harmed by these medications in utero. According to an FDA update
issued in June, 2009, "To provide information regarding the effects of
in utero exposure to Depakote, physicians are advised to recommend
that pregnant patients taking Depakote enroll in the North American

Antiepileptic Drug (NAAED) Pregnancy Registry. This can be done by calling the toll free number 1-888-233-2334, and must be done by patients themselves." Information on the registry can also be found on Massachusetts General Hospital's website, www.massgeneral.org.

Headaches After Childbirth and in the Postpartum Period

It is not uncommon to experience a return of headaches within a week or two following delivery. For headache-prone women, it may be best be proactive about discussing headache management as part of your "postpartum care," even before birth. Headaches that develop immediately following giving birth or during the first few weeks of the postpartum period may occur for a variety of reasons. In an article addressed to healthcare providers entitled, *Postpartum Headache—Is Your Workup Complete*, by physicians at the University of Cincinnati College of Medicine, experts reviewed the cases of 95 women who experienced severe headache at least 24 hours or more after giving birth, ranging from 2 to 32 days, with a mean onset of 3 to 4 days. Major causes of headache included preeclampsia or eclampsia (in 24% of cases), dural puncture from anesthesia (16%), and neurological lesions. However, the majority of postpartum headaches (47%) were primary headaches, diagnosed as either TTH or migraine.

Twenty-two cases of the 95 patients studied had neurological symptoms or failed to respond to conservative therapies, and cerebral imaging showed that 15 of these women had abnormal findings. Ten women had serious cerebral pathologies, including bleeding in the brain or blood clots, leading researchers to develop a step-by-step, multidisciplinary protocol for evaluating women with serious postpartum headaches. The recommendations include:

- The possibility of preeclampsia should be considered in women with high blood pressure and protein in their urine, indicating kidney dysfunction; women without these findings should be evaluated first for TTH, or if appropriate, low-pressure spinal headache.
- Women with headaches that are unresponsive to usual treatments or that are accompanied by neurological symptoms require imaging to rule out potentially life-threatening causes.

These serious complications related to postpartum headache have specific treatments that are well beyond the scope of this book. But the point is, not all postpartum headaches are benign, or harmless, and there are protocols to follow carefully before excluding these serious health conditions. A large study of women with migraines showed little evidence that breastfeeding has any negative effect on headaches, but just as in pregnancy, you will need to continue to avoid most medications while breast-feeding and make use of alternative methods when possible. With your physician's guidance, you may be able to use Imitrex (sumatriptan) in injection form during breastfeeding, but some researchers feel that more study is needed for its use in pregnancy. If you suffer from problem headaches, have a discussion with your physician, preferably before becoming pregnant.

Headache During Peri-Menopause and Menopause

For some women who rarely experienced hormonal headaches during their reproductive years, peri-menopause and menopause seem to bring on headaches; this is likely due to the erratic fluctuations in the hormones that trigger migraines. Other women simply continue to experience headaches after menopause; if headaches remain after menopause, your usual medications and lifestyle modifications can help to manage your symptoms. You may also want to speak to your OB/GYN about using supplemental, bioidentical estrogen to manage both your headaches and the other bothersome symptoms of menopause such as hot flashes and irritability. A low, steady supply of estrogen is best for helping to prevent estrogen-withdrawal headaches. One effective way to achieve this is to use estrogen in a patch application, changing it two to three times per week.

Women face special challenges in dealing with headaches through the lifespan. We're all unique, which means that the prevention, diagnosis and treatment of headaches must be tailored to each of us as individuals. A one-size-fits-all approach rarely works, whether in clothing size or headache management.

The next chapter examines what happens when headaches begin to occur very frequently and what steps can be taken to help manage, or alleviate, chronic headaches.

Chronic Daily Headaches

I've done a lot of research on chronic daily headaches during the two and a half years that I suffered from them. In some on-line forums, I've met people who have lived with CDH for 8, 10, even 20 years. Even with all the treatment options out there, there don't seem to be any magic bullets. It's a process of elimination, both in finding a practitioner who will treat you with respect and compassion, as well as in finding treatments that work for you. Some people have had great results with Botox, acupuncture, or with the selective calcium antagonist Sibelium. Some forms of chronic daily headache can be successfully managed with preventive medications. It's really important to give the medications you try time to work, which can take up to 2-3 months. Often, it's a combination of treatments and medications that seem to help the most. Be careful to avoid OTC medications and narcotics, as they can cause rebound headaches. Watch out for the depression and anxiety that can result from suffering debilitating headaches on a daily or near-daily basis. You also need to do your own investigation and learn to ask the right questions about your own body. Does your pain increase when you cough or bend over? Do you have other physical ailments, like fibromyalgia or chronic fatigue, allergies, asthma, or gastrointestinal problems? Did your headache pattern set in after a traumatic accident or a surgery gone wrong? These may be indicators of which direction you need to look for answers. And maybe your answers do not lie in ever- better medications, but in a careful effort to eliminate environmental and food triggers, trying stress reduction practices like yoga or chi gong, and focusing on your overall health. Keep an open mind and never give up hope that your condition will improve. Thankfully, my headaches responded to a holistic approach, and now I only have to deal with an occasional migraine. Suffering from a headache that builds up every single day is only a nightmare from the past. SAMANTHA

The World Health Organization reports that up to 1 in 20 adults has a headache every day, or nearly every day, and that chronic daily headache is a significant global problem. Chronic daily headache (CDH) is defined as headache occurring more than 15 days per month, each lasting for more than 4 hours. To meet the official criteria for diagnosis for primary CDH, this condition must have persisted for at least 3 months and there must not be an identifiable infectious or structural cause. Overall, CDH may affect as many as 5% of the population, although some authorities feel this figure is low and consider CDH to be one of the most prevalent headache disorders in the United States. Why the discrepancy? Because many CDH sufferers routinely self-medicate with over-the-counter (OTC) analgesics and are not receiving medical care through which they might be counted in prevalence estimates. Curiously, the condition seems to occur most often in two age groups—those in their early 20s and people over the age of 64.

Types of Primary Chronic Daily Headaches

Two of the most common primary types of CDH are chronic migraine (CM) and chronic tension-type headache (CTTH). CTTH is present in 2% to 3% of the population and CM affects about 2%. Some people can have combined tension and migraine headaches, or "mixed headache," with features of both CTTH and CM.

Chronic TTH is much more disabling than episodic TTH, from which it evolves. CTTH must cause mild-to-moderate pain on both sides of the head, but without the pulsating, throbbing quality of migraine. The symptoms of CTTH are not aggravated by normal physical activity and they do not generally involve the same degree of sensitivity to light or sound as migraine. If nausea is present, it is mild and very rarely leads to vomiting. Symptoms may wax and wane or may have a more constant presence. Headaches frequently begin in the occipital region (back of the head) and the muscles that run up the back of the neck may be unusually tense, or even tender. Current diagnostic criteria for CTTH require TTH headache on at least 15 days a month for 3 months, but they do not specify the number of hours of headache duration.

The CM was formerly called "transformed migraine," and it is thought to evolve or "transform" from episodic migraine without aura. Beyond the pain of migraine headache, CM also requires two of these additional symptoms on at least 8 days each month: one-sided location, pulsating pain, and worsening with physical activity. Either nausea or vomiting, or sensitivity to light or sound must also be present. Positive response to triptans or ergot-based medications helps to confirm the diagnosis of CM.

According to headache expert Dr. Stephen D. Silberstein, the most recent International Classification of Headache Disorders-II (ICHD-II) algorithm classifies CM as a "complication of migraine." Diagnostic criteria are migraine headache occurring on 15 or more days a month for more than 3 months, but medication overuse must first be ruled out, or if present, the medication must have been withdrawn completely for at least 2 months. Episodic migraine headache is also usually present in an individual prior to the onset of CM.

Two other primary forms of CDH, Chronic Cluster Headache (CCH) and Hemicrania continua (HC) are discussed in Chapter 12—Trigeminal Autonomic Cephalgias. The Mayo Clinic and other sources list some possible factors that may contribute to primary CDH, including the following:

- Chronic stress—a risk factor in many headache types, and definitely in CDH. Many patients also suffer from anxiety or depression.
- Overuse of OTC and prescription pain relievers in headache treatment.

- The development of a heightened response to pain signals (see Chapter 1).
- Obesity—in a study involving over 1,000 chronic headache sufferers, it was found that people who are obese have about *twice* the incidence of CDH as those of healthier weight.
- The use of caffeine, alcohol, and tobacco.
- Poor sleep, including snoring and sleep apnea; people with CDH are more likely to suffer from these problems than nonheadache sufferers.
- Poor posture that leads to chronic neck strain is another risk factor, which was discussed in Chapter 2.

Types of Secondary Chronic Headaches

Secondary CDH is related to the existence of an underlying medical disorder. Several of these headaches will be discussed in later chapters of the book, which covers secondary headaches. New Daily Persistent Headache (NDPH), a secondary CDH type recently added to the ICHD-II classification, is discussed in Chapter 16. NDPH affects far fewer people than CTTH or CM. Some possible causes of secondary CDH are listed below:

- Uncontrolled systemic inflammation in the body, which can affect blood vessels in the brain.
- An imbalance in intracranial pressure—either too high (idiopathic intracranial hypertension) or too low (idiopathic intracranial

What Nurses Know...

Medication overuse, stress, poor sleep, obesity, cigarette smoking, and the overuse of caffeine and alcohol are the key "modifiable risk factors," meaning that we have the power to make positive changes in these lifestyle factors—and doing so may help to eliminate chronic daily headaches.

hypotension)—sometimes related to an excess of cerebrospinal fluid (CSF) or the surgical treatment for this condition, or to unrelated factors.

- When CDH is due to low pressure it may be called "low pressure headache." The headache is felt most severely after sitting upright, and lessens when lying down. Low pressure headaches are caused by the leakage of CSF. CSF leaks can occur spontaneously, due to injury, or as the result of accidental puncture of the dural membrane when placing a catheter for epidural anesthesia for childbirth or postsurgery pain relief, or as the result of a spinal tap. These headaches can sometimes be repaired by placing a tiny amount of the patient's own blood into the epidural space, called an "epidural blood patch" (EBP).
- Posttraumatic headache due to traumatic brain injury; although past studies have been inconsistent, we are now beginning to learn more about the relationship between head and neck injury and CDH (see Chapter 14—Head Injury-Related Headaches).
- The presence of an underlying infection.
- Chronic musculoskeletal pain disorders, including arthritis.
- Overuse of OTC or prescription pain relievers.

The overuse of OTC or prescription pain relievers is present in approximately 30% of people who suffer from CDH. Obviously, proper use of medications is something that needs to be closely monitored.

MEDICATION OVERUSE HEADACHE

In essence, medication overuse headache develops when susceptible patients overuse pain-relieving medications, defined as more frequently than 10 to 15 days per month, without going for long periods of time without medication. Medication overuse headache (MOH) subtypes are based on headaches in relation to various classes of medications. For neurologists as well as patients, the overuse of pain-relieving medications greatly complicates the accurate diagnosis of true CDH, and the possibility of MOH must be ruled out before diagnosing other chronic headache disorders. There may be a central nervous system mechanism that plays a role in MOH because such "rebound" headaches have been known to occur with a wide range of medications including the following:

- Caffeine and medications containing caffeine
- Ergotamine and other ergot-derived drugs
- Opiates
- OTC analgesics and antiinflammatories some prescription headache medications
- Triptans (although this is still under debate)

MOH tends to be constant and unremitting, with the possible exception of headaches associated with triptans, which may be more intermittent. Patients taking opioids tend to have the highest relapse rate following treatment for MOH.

Among patients who seek treatment for CDH at specialty clinics, about 80% have a history of medication overuse. A closely supervised medication-withdrawal program aided by preventive medications can lead to reduced headache frequency in many, but not all, patients. Patients should not attempt to do this on their own, as serious side effects can occur, including: a temporary worsening of headache, excessive sweating, agitation, and less commonly—seizures. All changes in prescription drug use must be guided by your physician, but it may be safe to slowly taper off OTC analgesics by reducing your dose by one tablet per week. You should also make every effort to avoid

What Nurses Know...

Studies have shown that it isn't always clear what is primarily responsible for successful resolution of CDH—medication withdrawal, or, the effects of newly added preventive drugs or other treatments. The entire withdrawal process can take as long as two months before the effects are clear, but once your headache frequency is significantly reduced you may notice that any episodic headaches will respond much better to your acute headache medications.

activities that trigger or worsen your headaches during this time, and be sure to drink plenty of fluids and get sufficient rest.

CHRONIC DAILY HEADACHE AND HEAD TRAUMA

Traumatic brain injury (TBI) is also called postconcussive syndrome (PCS) and is discussed under secondary headache types in Chapter 14. But it is important to note that posttraumatic headache is an important, and increasing, subtype of CDH. Many members of the armed forces are returning from active duty in the Middle East with headaches that are the result of head trauma. Repeatedly suffering even minor head trauma from explosions, gunfire, vehicle accidents, and blows to the head adds up—unfortunately, to CDH.

Seeking Help for Chronic Daily Headache

Seeing your primary care physician is a good place to start. You may be referred to a neurologist or headache specialist right away, or after examining you and collecting your headache history, your doctor may feel comfortable developing an initial treatment plan. But, if your headaches do not respond after a few weeks, or worsen, ask for a referral to a specialist. Most doctors like to trial headache medications at least 2 months, but CDHs can be very difficult to

What Nurses Know...

Keeping a headache diary is an important aid to diagnosis in any headache type, but in CDH, it's essential. By definition, you need to meet specific criteria regarding the number of headache days, duration of headaches, and specific symptoms that help to narrow the diagnosis to the particular headache type. Include any non-headache symptoms, any medications or other treatments you've attempted, and any lifestyle or stress-related factors that may play a role in headaches.

manage and may be beyond your primary care doctor's expertise or resources.

DIAGNOSIS OF CHRONIC DAILY HEADACHE

Beyond the physical and neurological doctor's exam, other tests may be done to rule out systemic inflammatory disorders or infectious disease. Imaging studies including CT and MRI may be done to exclude any abnormalities within your brain that could be causing your headaches.

TREATMENT OF CHRONIC DAILY HEADACHE

With CDH, it is important to identify and avoid activities that make your headache pain worse. Try not to use your usual OTC pain relievers more than two or three times a week, as this increases the risk of MOH. You may be expecting to find a list of medications to treat acute symptoms here, but medications such as triptans are not designed for daily use. Many medications used to treat migraine and related headaches, including triptans, are vasoconstricting—and using them on a daily or near-daily basis may not be safe, especially for those with cardiac risk factors. So, seeking help from a headache specialist may lead to a more intense focus on prevention, using lifestyle changes, physical therapy or massage, and prophylactic medications. In Chapter 17, you will read about some new medications under development that may be safer for people who cannot take vasoconstricting medications.

CM is very difficult to treat and typically does not respond well to the usual migraine medications. It is possible that years of frequent CMs lead to permanent changes in the brain. Even if this is the case, there are treatments that can help to reduce pain and improve quality of life. But the *key* is to seek treatment as soon as it becomes clear that your headaches are becoming a problem, and work with your doctor to develop a preventive strategy as soon as possible. These actions may help to prevent the kinds of long-term changes that lead to treatment-resistant, intractable headaches.

An ever-present question is what causes the transformation from episodic or occasional to chronic headaches. For example, at least a third of CM patients seen in specialty headache clinics previously suffered only occasional migraine attacks. If pharmaceutical researchers and other scientists can learn to prevent this transformation, then the frustration of CDHs for both patients and their medical team can be greatly decreased.

CDH is actually fairly common, especially in women and in people suffering from chronic stress. Some headache experts believe that the ICHD-II diagnostic criteria of 15 headaches per month may not be set in stone, and that there may be subtypes of CDH with slightly different presentations.

PREVENTION

A variety of medications are used to prevent CDH, including tricyclic antidepressants like Pamelor (nortriptyline) or selective serotonin reuptake inhibitor (SSRI) antidepressants such as Prozac (fluoxetine). Beta-blockers such as atenolol or metoprolol may be effective, and may work well in combination with antidepressants. Anticonvulsants like Neurontin (gabapentin), Depakote (valproic acid derivatives), or Topamax (topiramate) may be used as well, although there are significant side effects to these medications. Their use in children is considered "off label," and neither Topamax nor Depakote can be used by women who are pregnant or are planning to become pregnant.

What Nurses Know...

GETTING HELP FOR CHRONIC HEADACHES

There are some simple indicators that you need to seek professional help for chronic headaches. See your doctor if you:

- *Have two or more headaches a week*
- *Take OTC or prescription pain relievers daily, or nearly every day*
- *If you feel you need to exceed the recommended dose of OTC medications to manage your headaches*
- *Your headaches seem to be changing or getting worse, or do not respond to rest and medication*

For those with CTTHs, Elavil is sometimes prescribed in doses of 10 to 75 mg. It is often taken prior to bedtime, as it can be sedating. Double-blind studies have confirmed its effectiveness in preventing CTTH, but side effects including blurred vision, hypotension, and weight gain may limit its use. Although one study showed that Prozac was nearly as effective as Amitriptyline, it took roughly two months to achieve the desired effect.

Nonsteroidal antiinflammatory drugs (NSAIDs) should be used very cautiously and not on a daily or near-daily basis, due to the risk of gastrointestinal side effects, as well as the more-recently discovered risk of heart arrhythmias. They are best saved for "break-through pain," or pain that occurs occasionally despite taking your usual medications. All NSAIDs should be taken with food and a full glass of liquid.

Trigger-point injections using local anesthetics combined with a corticosteroid may be used for CDH. And just recently, the use of Botox (botulinum toxin) injections has been approved for the treatment of CM. Botox injections have proven to be effective in treating migraine and CDH in the general population, in patients with whiplash neck injuries, and in soldiers with posttraumatic headache. Botox reduces muscle hyperactivity, which leads to decreased muscle tension. Research has suggested that Botox may provide central nervous system or antiinflammatory effects that may also help in the treatment of headaches, but the evidence is not yet definitive. Despite some controversy, studies suggest that Botox is safe, and one clear advantage is that it does not cause the systemic side effects associated with many other medications.

Occipital nerve stimulation, discussed in the treatment of cluster headache in Chapter 12, is an investigational treatment for CDH.

Headaches that prove resistant to conventional treatment may respond to complementary and alternative medicine (CAM) therapies, which are discussed in Chapter 5. Acupuncture, biofeedback, relaxation and stress-reduction techniques, and therapeutic massage may be of benefit in CDH treatment. In addition, some of the herbs and nutraceuticals used in migraine headache may be useful in reducing headache severity. These treatments include:

- Vitamin B2
- Magnesium
- Coenzyme Q10

The herbs feverfew and butterbur may be helpful, but they cannot be used in pregnancy. Relaxation, meditation, and biofeedback have proven to be very useful in treating CDH.

We've already discussed headache risk factors and headache triggers, both generally and in the treatment of TTH, migraine, and cluster headache. Discovering your specific triggers is a key to success. Making positive lifestyle changes involving diet, stress reduction, and maintaining healthy weight is very important. Equally so is getting moderate exercise at least three times a week, and enjoying sufficient restful sleep regularly. But regarding CDH, studies have shown clear associations between three other modifiable risk factors: the use of caffeine, alcohol, and tobacco. Think before you drink or smoke.

SUPPORT FOR COPING WITH CHRONIC PAIN

Coping with any type of chronic pain is very challenging to patients. Hopefully, you will respond well to the treatment offered by your healthcare team, and your headaches will decrease in both frequency and severity. During this transitional time of healing, many patients find it helpful to attend a support group. Various national headache organizations maintain a list of groups which headache patients can attend locally. They are listed in Chapter 18. Professional counseling with a therapist specializing in chronic pain is another option for getting the support you need. This might also be useful if you suffer from the severe, stabbing, headaches discussed in the next chapter.

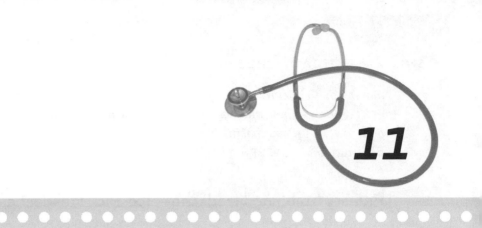

Primary Stabbing Headache (Idiopathic Stabbing Headache, Ice-Pick Headache)

Several members of my family suffer from ice-pick headaches. Usually located behind or around the ear, these headaches feel like someone is slipping an ice-pick under the skin for a second or two. There seems to be no direct trigger. I feel a very intense stab (the ice-pick label really fits!) always into the same spot on the left side of my head, and I really feel like I'm about to black out—then it's gone. If you have these headaches you will know it! They come out of nowhere any time day or night, last several seconds then disappear. CT and MRI scans show nothing. When they started waking me up out of sound sleep and I began having more than 5 or 6 attacks a day my doctor suggested amitriptyline, and I have found that it helps. It's not a cure, and it takes about two

months or so to start working, so don't give up if your headaches
don't improve immediately. Some members of my family have
done well on indomethacin, which works much more quickly than
amitriptyline.   STEVEN

Primary Stabbing Headache—"Ice-Pick Headache"

This startling, severe, headache is aptly named. People have been
known to fall to the ground when struck with the stabbing pain of an
ice-pick headache, which can come as a single stab or a series of quick
stabs. Many people have awakened abruptly in the early hours before
dawn with sudden pain in the temple, behind the ear, or surrounding
the eye. On a day when icepick headaches strike, an individual may
suffer *multiple attacks*. The odd thing about these headaches is that
they don't last long, often just a few excruciating moments (5–30 seconds). The ICHD-II classification criteria describe Primary Stabbing
Headache as "Transient and localized stabs of pain in the head that
occur spontaneously in the absence of organic disease of underlying
structures or of the cranial nerves." Stabbing headaches may occur
by themselves but they are more common in patients with other headaches like cluster and migraine. The National Institutes of Health
reports that as many as 40% of migraine patients have also suffered
an ice-pick headache, often on the same side as their migraines usually occur.

Due to their very short duration, primary stabbing headaches
may be underdiagnosed and more common than previously thought.

What Nurses Know...

These headaches belong to the group of "indomethacin-
responsive headaches"–primary headaches which are usu-
ally characterized by a rapid response and complete recovery
when treated with the drug indomethacin, but that are usu-
ally unresponsive to other NSAIDs or other medications used
to treat headache disorders.

Dr. Christina Peterson, a headache specialist in Portland, Oregon, relates that primary stabbing headache patients now make up a significant proportion of her practice. Ice-pick headache has also been called "jabs and jolts syndrome."

WHO GETS THEM AND WHY?

As with other primary headaches, ice-pick headaches don't appear to have an identifiable underlying cause, but there does seem to be an association with stress. Some researchers suspect sudden, transient changes in blood flow to certain areas of the brain—but what causes this to happen so abruptly is unknown. These headaches have a later age of onset than some other primary headaches—in the late 40's, although some people say their headaches began in childhood. In contrast to cluster headaches, ice-pick headaches tend to affect more women than men.

SYMPTOMS

Attacks of ice-pick headache may occur from once a day to an extreme of nearly 50 per day. Pain is usually felt along the distribution of the first branch of the trigeminal nerve, in the eye socket, temple, above the ears, and across the top of the head, and it is not usually accompanied by visual or other symptoms as in migraine. Occasionally, there may be some nausea, vertigo, tearing, runny nose, or reddened eyes associated with ice-pick headache, but these symptoms are less prominent than with headaches in the Trigeminal Autonomic Cephalgias/cluster headache group. Some ice-pick headache sufferers report that the intensity of pain is worsened by bright light or movement during an attack. But the most characteristic symptoms of ice-pick headache are the suddenness of the attack and its brevity. In fact, the pain is so abrupt and severe that some patients may fear they've had a TIA, stroke, or ruptured aneurysm, and in a first attack, it's very hard for any patient to know the difference.

DIAGNOSIS

As with other primary headache types, diagnosis depends on an accurate and complete patient headache history. It's best to record the

What Nurses Know...

A TIA, or mini-stroke, is the result of an arterial clot disrupting blood flow to the brain, depriving brain tissues of oxygen. A TIA causes neurological symptoms such as numbness, tingling, problems with speech or vision, and difficulties with balance, but it typically causes no head pain. Only a small fraction of headaches are related to a more serious vascular problem in the brain, like a clot or a ruptured aneurysm.

experience in a headache diary in detail and to follow up with a physician as soon as possible to obtain an accurate diagnosis. Be sure to include the time of headache onset, length of headache, what you were doing at the time, and what helps provide relief or aggravates your symptoms. (Finding effective relief measures may be difficult to do given the brief nature of ice-pick headache.) Your physician then will do a thorough physical and neurological exam and may order diagnostic imaging or other tests to rule out other conditions which could create similar symptoms. This is especially important in primary stabbing headache. Anyone experiencing a first episode of sudden onset, stabbing head pain should not assume it is ice-pick headache. It may instead be a much more serious, even life-threatening, condition such as a stroke or rupture of a brain aneurysm.

Sudden intense headaches can come from a variety of sources including eating something very cold too quickly—the dreaded-but-harmless "ice cream headache." A sudden pulsing, throbbing headache may also result from carbon monoxide poisoning or from exposure to toxic chemicals like solvents—in these cases a sudden, bad headache is a sign that the body is suffering from systemic poisoning that can lead to organ failure, permanent neurological damage, or even death. The body is "sounding the alarm," and it should never be ignored. In pregnant women, a sudden bad headache can be a sign of preeclampsia or toxemia, which can lead to very high blood pressure that poses a danger to the mother and the fetus—and it requires immediate medical attention. An unusual cause of a sudden bad headache is the overuse of decongestant nasal sprays containing oxymetazoline, which can cause rapid constriction or narrowing of blood vessels in the brain. Discontinuing use of the medicated nasal spray usually relieves the headache.

TREATMENT

Treatment of ice-pick headaches is difficult, because it is impossible to predict when they will occur and the episodes of acute pain are so brief. But in those people with frequent, recurring ice-pick headaches, the NSAID Indocin (indomethacin) is sometimes used, and is effective in about 65% of patients. Therapy is started with a low dose and tapered up until headaches decrease in frequency and severity, usually at about 25-50 mg of indomethacin per day—for adults. Side effects of indomethacin include various gastrointestinal complaints, bleeding problems, and less frequently, redness, yellowing, or blurring of vision. So anyone taking indomethacin should receive regular eye exams, and seek immediate help if blurred vision occurs while on indomethacin. Indomethacin cannot be taken by people with kidney disease or by people taking blood-thinning medications. Long-term use of indomethacin has been linked to increased risk of heart attack or stroke.

Beta-blockers, drugs used to treat high blood pressure and angina, may be another option for some patients. Other medications used to treat ice-pick headaches include tricyclic antidepressants and anticonvulsant medications.

The hormone melatonin, produced by the pineal gland, has been used in a few case studies as a successful ice-pick headache treatment. Melatonin helps to regulate sleep and inflammation. Based on three documented case reports published in the journal *Neurology*, melatonin helped to relieve ice-pick headaches at doses varying from 3 to 12 mg daily, taken at bedtime. Two of the three patients had been unable to tolerate indomethacin but responded well to melatonin. All three patients remained headache-pain free after a minimum of two months of continued melatonin. In a small study of adults with ice-pick headaches patients were treated with an oral dose of 3 mg of melatonin every night for 6 months, then melatonin was withdrawn for 6 months. The study's results were encouraging. You can discuss this possibility with your doctor.

As an alternate treatment for indomethacin, melatonin is important because it has relatively few serious side effects or other drug interactions. Interestingly, this hormone has a chemical structure that is similar to the NSAID indomethacin. There is some evidence that supplemental melatonin can lower seizure threshold, especially in children, but this possible risk remains controversial. Certainly anyone with a history of seizure should not self-medicate, and if taking prescribed melatonin, should be closely followed by a physician. Side effects of melatonin can include the following:

- Fatigue
- Dizziness
- Mood changes
- A feeling of being "hung over" in the morning

Side-effects occur especially if the dose is too high. Melatonin is not recommended for women who are pregnant or nursing. Increased risks of bleeding and lowered blood pressure have also been reported. Because it causes drowsiness, melatonin should be taken at bedtime, and in fact, melatonin is often prescribed as a sleep aid. It's important to use caution and inform your physician before taking any new medications, whether they're prescription, OTC, or "nutraceuticals."

Magnesium deficiency has been suggested as a factor in migraine and certainly studies have shown supplemental magnesium to be of benefit for many patients. I was not able to find a similar connection between ice-pick headaches and magnesium supplementation, but it may be worth trying the recommended dose of an OTC magnesium supplement if you are desperate for relief. Magnesium is helpful in many other conditions involving vasoconstriction.

Some patients with ice-pick headache say they have benefitted from acupuncture. Other complementary therapies include relaxation and deep breathing, which can help you to get through an attack of ice-pick headache pain without panicking. As with other severe headaches that come on suddenly (including cluster and related headaches, discussed in the next chapter), always put your own safety, as well as the safety of those around you, first if you feel even a twinge of an oncoming attack.

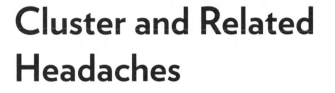

Cluster and Related Headaches

I am a sixty-year-old male, who has suffered from cluster head aches for the past 10 years, usually during the summer months. I awake in the middle of the night to a piercing pain originating on the upper right side of my skull, accompanied by mild tearing in my right eye, and the contraction of my right iris. The pain is almost unbearable for about 45 minutes and then it gradually subsides, but it usually takes another thirty to sixty minutes before I can fall asleep again. This disruption of my normal sleep pattern is a significant side effect of the headaches, causing reduced productivity during the workday. My neurologist has discussed pharmaceutical pain management options with me, but I choose not to use these drugs. Instead, I place an ice cube between my upper and lower teeth, directly below the spot in my head where the pain originates, softly biting the ice until it melts. I usually work my way through four or five ice cubes, while the cold numbs the pain and provides a limited amount of relief. The consistency of the pain pattern and the fact that my

*headaches occur for only a few weeks each year have taught me
that I can and will survive this challenging medical condition.
I know that my headaches will come and go, and I have learned
to live with them.* BILL

This group of headaches shares some common characteristics: one-sided location, eye-related symptoms such as tearing, and the intensity with which they strike. But one of the most distinctive aspects of "trigeminal autonomic cephalgias" as a group is that they share symptoms controlled by the autonomic nervous system—which is responsible for control of the body's involuntary actions including intestinal, cardiovascular, and endocrine functions. The three disorders discussed in this category include cluster headache, paroxysmal hemicranias, and short-lasting unilateral neuralgiform headache attacks with conjunctival tearing (abbreviated SUNCT).

Cluster Headaches: Who Gets Them and Why?

Cluster headaches affect far fewer individuals than do tension-type headaches or migraines, but because the pain is so severe patients with cluster headache may be more likely to seek medical treatment than those with other primary headache types. These "clusters" of short-duration headaches occur in just over 1-in-1000 individuals and they tend to affect more men than women, although there is not as much gender disparity as was previously thought. Chronic cluster headache, which is very rare, does affect a much larger proportion of men.

People usually begin to experience cluster headaches in their late twenties to early thirties and continue to experience them through mid-life. Cluster headaches can also be found in children. Like migraine, there appears to be some genetic basis for cluster headaches: Studies conducted with identical twins and with close relatives of cluster headache patients indicate that these headaches are found with far greater frequency in family members than would be expected. There is an overlap with migraine headache, with a small percentage of migraine sufferers also experiencing cluster headaches.

Many cluster headache patients describe a seasonal or climate-related association, with most headache clusters occurring in the spring or fall. There is also regularity to the start and duration of each cluster period, which often lasts from 6 to 12 weeks. During a cluster period, consuming certain foods may trigger an attack, while these same foods may not be problematic outside of the cluster period. Dietary triggers include: foods high in tyramine; nitrites and nitrates found in preserved meats; and foods containing MSG. Cluster headaches are sometimes called "histamine headaches," and certainly some foods high in histamines, such as red wine, also seem to trigger headaches during a cluster period. Studies have also shown that in 69% of patients, subcutaneous histamine injection will provoke an attack. But research on the exact nature of the role of histamines is inconsistent, and unfortunately, antihistamines do not prevent or alleviate acute cluster headaches. It's possible that cluster attacks may also be triggered by other conditions that promote histamine release, such as stress, chronic inflammation, and exposure to food and environmental allergens.

An association between alcohol use and cluster headaches is well documented, with 50% of patients having a history of heavy alcohol use. Smoking is another huge risk factor, with more than 80% of cluster headache patients being heavy smokers. Exposure to volatile solvents and high altitude travel are some other common triggers for cluster headache.

Symptoms

Cluster headaches most often strike without warning, causing sufferers excruciating pain that quickly reaches a peak within 5 to 10 minutes. Cluster headaches take their name from their tendency to strike on multiple occasions in a discrete period of time, in attacks lasting from a few minutes to a few hours. Attacks often begin in the late evening or a few hours after bedtime—a time when it is common for people to enter the first period of sleep known as REM (rapid eye movement). The number of attacks can vary from a single daily attack to many attacks within one day. In most patients this "cluster" of headaches is followed by a period of remission sometimes lasting as long as several years, during which no headaches occur. Unfortunately, in about 10% of cases, cluster headaches can become chronic. In both episodic and chronic cluster headaches, symptom severity causes patients to miss work, educational and social opportunities, and other important aspects of life, which can lead to depression and a feeling of hopelessness.

People with these unusually intense headaches describe recurrent attacks of burning, searing pain localized to one side of the head, usually behind or surrounding the eye, or in the temple area, although pain can also radiate to adjacent areas of the face, head, and neck. Often the affected eyelid will appear to be reddened, swollen, and slightly drooping, the pupil will be constricted, and there will be tearing of the eye. Sometimes these signs are accompanied by nasal congestion or a runny nose, and the face may feel moist or clammy, signs of autonomic nervous system involvement. Less frequently, patients may have increased sweating of the upper body in general. There may be acute scalp and facial tenderness which recedes when the headache resolves. It is important to note, though, that touch does not actually provoke pain in the case of cluster headache, as it does in the facial pain disorder trigeminal neuralgia (TN).

In contrast to many migraine patients, who often want only to lie down in a dark room, the pain of cluster headaches is agitating, causing restlessness and a need for motor activities such as walking, pacing, or rocking back and forth. This restlessness affects about 90% of patients with cluster headaches. Some have even been known to hurt themselves by scratching or rubbing at the locus of the pain in the forehead or surrounding the eye. For people with cluster headaches, lying down seems to worsen symptoms, rather than helping to alleviate them, a significant difference from many other headache types.

In research studies, PET scans of people with cluster headaches show areas of increased blood flow in part of the hypothalamus, located deep within the brain. This increased blood flow occurs only on the side where the headache is felt. The hypothalamus is a part of our endocrine system that plays a vital role in regulating the autonomic nervous system—which in turn controls the body fluid secretion and blood vessel changes that accompany cluster headaches. The hypothalamus also governs our internal biological clock, which is consistent with the cyclical nature of cluster headache, and the fact that headaches tend to occur at the same time each day.

The complete biochemical picture of cluster headaches is still somewhat of a mystery but it may involve activation of nerve cells along the first and second divisions of the trigeminal nerve. The branched trigeminal nerve is the largest cranial nerve and the major sensory nerve in the face. It is involved in the production of temperature and pain signals and in relaying this information to the brain. The activated trigeminal nerve is responsible for the eye pain associated with cluster headaches, and by stimulating different nerves, the trigeminal nerve is indirectly responsible for eye-related symptoms such as redness and tearing, and autonomic nervous symptoms such as facial sweating.

As in migraine, the vascular changes seen in cluster headache are thought to be secondary to nerve activation and the release of Substance P and other inflammatory neurotransmitters that carry sensory and motor impulses to the affected nerves. Other similarities to migraine include occasional sensitivity to light and sound affecting only one side of the head and face. Aura may be present in about 14% of patients, but it is usually less pronounced than in migraine.

There may be some subtle signs that a cluster headache is imminent, including a mild discomfort or burning behind one eye, or sweating and flushing of one side of the forehead or temple. Sensitivity to light may increase. Other eye-related symptoms usually begin with the headache.

Diagnosis

After ruling out other conditions which can cause neurological symptoms, diagnosis is based on a detailed patient history involving repeated attacks with a clustering pattern. ICHD-II diagnostic criteria state that patients must have at least five attacks occurring in a frequency from every other day up to eight headaches per day and that there must be no other obvious cause for headaches. To distinguish between episodic cluster headache and chronic cluster headache, a headache-free period lasting at least one month is required. In chronic cluster headache, the remission period is less than one month. Imaging is not required to diagnose cluster headache, but a CT scan or MRI may be used to rule out other serious causes of head pain if the neurological exam is abnormal.

The cause of cluster headaches has not yet been identified but the associated pain is thought to result from the sudden dilation of pain-sensitive blood vessels. Cluster headache can be evoked by the drug nitroglycerine, and experimentally, by the administration of nitric oxide—a molecule that activates nerve pathways and helps to regulate arterial blood flow. Either increased nitric oxide production or hyper-responsiveness to nitric oxide may play a part in triggering both migraines and cluster headache by triggering inflammation and hyperactivity along the affected trigeminal nerve pathways.

Treatment

The pain of cluster headache is so severe that it is important to have a rescue strategy, whether it is going to lie in a dark room with an icepack, taking OTC medications, or using prescription medications. Many emergency room physicians have found that having patients inhale 100% oxygen by mask at 7 liters/minute is effective in alleviating most cluster headaches within 15 to 20 minutes, especially if used quickly after headache onset. But in everyday life this treatment can be impractical for some people. Although oral use of Imitrex (sumatriptan) is not found to be effective in aborting cluster headache, sumatriptan by injection is more effective. In many cases, patients can be taught to give their own subcutaneous injections using a tiny, short needle similar to the process used in self-injecting insulin. And two recent research studies show that zolmitriptan, or zomig, which can be administered as a nasal spray, may reduce the pain of cluster headaches within 10 to 30 minutes; the spray was effective at both the 5 and 10 mg doses. Dihydroergotamine (DHE, Migranal), a classic acute medication for cluster headaches, is available in injectable and inhaled forms. These medications may be effective treatments for some people, but ergot medications cannot be combined with triptans, and they are only for short-term use. Triptans and ergotamines are not recommended for people with uncontrolled high blood pressure or ischemic heart disease—cautions which are common with all vasoconstrictive medications. Octreotide (sandostatin, octreotide acetate) is a synthetic hormone that may be effective in alleviating cluster headache. It is considered safe for those with cardiovascular risk factors. Finally, another treatment offered is intranasal lidocaine (which can be applied with a swab), a local anesthetic that acts very quickly to reduce pain.

During a headache cluster period, or season, it may be important to take a medication to help prevent headache reoccurrence, especially if clusters usually last longer than a few weeks. With your physician's help, you may be able to taper off these medications when the cluster period ends, but do not stop taking any medication without your physician's guidance. There are many possible medications used to prevent cluster headaches:

- indomethacin
- verapamil
- lithium
- Depakote
- Topamax
- prednisone

Many of these medications can have significant side effects.

Short-term relief for cluster headache also includes administering nerve blocks. These may include a local anesthetic combined with a steroid, injected into the tissue surrounding the occipital nerve at the back of the head. The occipital nerve pathway intersects with the trigeminal nerve, which regulates the pain-sensitive tissues in the skull.

Newer treatments under investigation include deep brain stimulation of the hypothalamus and occipital nerve stimulation. Deep brain stimulation requires surgery to implant a small, impulse-emitting, electrode in close proximity to the hypothalamus—the region of the brain associated with the timing of cluster periods. The treatment has the potential to change the brain's electrical impulses and may help to alleviate the pain of cluster headache. Occipital nerve stimulation also involves implanting a small electrode in the back of the head. Stimulating the occipital nerve via electrical impulses may help to block pain signals. Initial studies have found these devices to be able to reduce chronic headache pain in some patients, and they appear to be well tolerated. These therapies are still in the experimental stages and may be most appropriate for patients with severe chronic cluster headaches. Rarely, other more aggressive surgical procedures usually focusing on the trigeminal nerve may be attempted for patients with unrelenting chronic cluster headaches—but the long-term benefits of such surgery has been questioned.

The Mayo Clinic reports that fewer than 10% of cluster headache patients were able to find lasting benefit from CAM therapies such as acupuncture, acupressure, therapeutic touch, chiropractic care, or homeopathy. However, several natural or herbal supplements do show some promise in reducing the intensity, frequency, and length of cluster headache attacks. An extract of the kudzu vine is one possibility being investigated. The Mayo Clinic also reports that 10 mg of the hormone melatonin taken in the evening may help to reduce the frequency of nighttime cluster attacks. Capsaicin, a pepper extract used as a nasal spray treatment to the affected side of the head, may help to decrease the frequency and severity of cluster headaches.

Prevention

It's impossible to prevent a first occurrence of cluster headache and once you begin to experience headaches it may take some time for your physician to accurately diagnose your headaches and prescribe treatment. You can help tremendously by keeping an accurate headache diary logging headache events and possible triggers, and also by continuing to document your headache-free periods. All patients can reduce headache risk by abstaining from alcohol, avoiding nicotine, and getting adequate restful sleep, especially during cluster periods. More than a decade ago, a British study demonstrated that increased body temperature may be a trigger for cluster headaches. It has been suggested that some patients can decrease the frequency of cluster headaches by maintaining a cool environment and avoiding hot baths and spas. Increased body heat can also be generated by exertion from exercise or sexual activity. This is not to say that these activities must be avoided! They are both healthy activities and important parts of a person's life. But staying well-hydrated and trying not to push the envelope too far may be important strategies for preventing cluster headaches.

Navigating life with cluster headache can be challenging for everyone. Even after a headache resolves, the fear of another headache attack can create tremendous anxiety. It may help to speak with a counselor in a chronic pain specialty clinic, or with a therapist who helps to treat those with chronic pain. Other options include joining a headache support group to meet others who truly understand what you are going through; support group members may be able to provide you with valuable information on health practitioners and other resources.

Paroxysmal Hemicranias and SUNCT

These unusual, unilateral headaches are considered to be rare variants of cluster headache. Both involve pain experienced along the affected trigeminal nerve pathways, and both are more common in women than men.

PAROXYSMAL HEMICRANIAS

The word "hemicrania" literally means "half the head." Paroxysmal hemicrania shares many characteristics with cluster headache, including tearing of the eye, nasal discharge, and other signs of autonomic nervous system involvement. Variations include *episodic* paroxysmal hemicrania and *chronic* paroxysmal hemicranias (CPH). About 90% of the time CPH occurs in women. CPH differs from cluster headache by having a shorter duration—each attack lasts only 5 to 30 minutes. But the attacks are "paroxysmal," occurring spontaneously up to 15 times per day, much more frequently than cluster headaches. The severe pain is much the same, though, affecting the eye, cheek, and temple on one side of the head.

HEMICRANIA CONTINUA

Hemicrania continua (HC) has similar clinical features, but one-sided moderate head and facial pain is present continuously and is punctuated by sudden episodes of sharper, short-lasting, stabbing pain. HC is sometimes responsive to indomethacin, as are many of the Trigeminal Autonomic Cephalgias headaches. The official classification criteria of HC include the following:

- Continuous, daily, one-sided headache present for three months, without pain-free periods.
- Moderate headache intensity with sharp exacerbations of more severe pain.

- At least one autonomic feature: tearing, nasal congestion or runny nose, drooping eyelid, or noticeable narrowing of the pupil on the same side as the headache.
- Headache is responsive to the therapeutic dose of the NSAID Indocin (indomethacin).

HC can also exist in a form that includes pain-free remissions lasting weeks to months. There is also a recognized variant of HC in which the headache meets the above diagnostic criteria but the affected side during an attack is not consistent and can shift.

Diagnosis follows the same process as in other headache types with the notable exception that "response to indomethacin" is considered diagnostic. HC is not usually responsive to triptans and other medications used in migraine or cluster headache. But in other ways, HC can resemble migraine, and can include throbbing pain, nausea, and vomiting, as well as sensitivity to light and sound. HC also may respond to Celebrex (celecoxib). But celecoxib carries an FDA-mandated "black box warning" for cardiovascular and gastrointestinal risk and in 2007, the American Heart Association posted this warning: "Celecoxib should be used as a last resort [for] patients who have heart disease or a risk of developing it." Celebrex should also not be used with alcohol or the anticoagulant drug Warfarin (Coumadin).

SUNCT

SUNCT stands for "Short-lasting, Unilateral, Neuralgiform headache attacks with Conjunctival injection and Tearing." That's a long, complicated term to describe one-sided headache attacks characterized by bursts of throbbing pain around the eye and temple. But these attacks last only 30 to 120 seconds or, rarely, up to 4 minutes!

SUNCT is more common in women, and attacks may be provoked by tactile stimulation or certain movements of the neck. This rare disorder may include a drooping eyelid and reddened, bloodshot eye, and it always features tearing as a symptom. The painful but brief attacks quickly ramp up to a peak and then subside. Unfortunately, an affected person may have up to six attacks per hour, which, if left untreated or resistant to treatment, makes normal life almost impossible.

TREATMENT

It can be difficult to distinguish between SUNCT and TN, but SUNCT does not usually respond to treatment with anticonvulsants, and the facial pain disorder TN often does. Neither SUNCT nor CPH respond to Imitrex. CPH is responsive to indomethacin (Indocin), which helps in distinguishing it from chronic migraine, while SUNCT is not. In fact, SUNCT responds poorly to many medications, but there are some recent reports of success using the anticonvulsants lamotrigine, topiramate, and gabapentin, and intravenous lidocaine. Two of the newest treatments to be investigated include the drug Zonegran (zonisamide), a sulfonamide anticonvulsant, and occipital nerve stimulation (discussed under cluster headache). Further research is underway.

Trigeminal Neuralgia

The word "neuralgia" simply means nerve pain, but it is defined as an intense, electric-shock-like pain felt along a specific nerve pathway and in the part of the body supplied by the affected nerve. Throughout the book I mention specific types of neuralgia, such as occipital neuralgia, or postherpetic neuraligia following a shingles outbreak. Trigeminal neuralgia (TN) is a condition caused by pain originating from the trigeminal nerve. This nerve carries pain, feeling, and other sensations from the brain to the skin of the face. It can affect part or all of the face as well as the surface of the eye. Because it shares so many similarities with the headaches discussed in this chapter, I've chosen to include it here for the purposes of comparison, especially because TN closely resembles SUNCT.

WHO GETS THEM AND WHY?

TN occurs most often in people over age 50, but it can occur at any age. It is more common in women than in men, and there is some evidence that the disorder runs in families. TN affects the trigeminal nerve, which supplies sensation to the face, causing daily attacks of intermittent severe burning pain lasting from thirty minutes to several hours. TN comes in clusters of attacks, similar to the pattern of cluster headache, and then subsides for an indefinite period of time, leaving patients with fear and anxiety regarding the next attack. TN may be caused by dilated blood vessels pulsating against the trigeminal nerve, or there may be some deterioration of the nerve's protective myelin sheath. This is suspected because TN also is found in some patients with MS. But most of the time the cause is unknown.

SYMPTOMS

The trigeminal nerve has three branches that conduct sensations from the upper, middle, and lower portions of the face and mouth to the brain. The upper branch supplies sensation to most of the scalp, forehead, and temples. The middle branch provides sensation to the cheek, upper jaw, top lip, teeth and gums, and side of the nose. The nerve's lower branch affects the lower jaw, teeth, gums, and bottom lip. TN can affect more than one of these nerve branches, and pain can be felt on only one side, or on both sides of the face, although not at the same time.

Some people experience a warning feeling a few days before an attack. This may be a tingling or numb sensation, or aching pain. Symptoms include headache and stabbing pain that comes on suddenly and is typically felt on one side of the jaw or cheek. Muscle spasms may occur on the affected side of the face. After the attack period begins, pain can be triggered by simple vibration, by light contact with the cheek or forehead from normal activities of daily living such as bathing, putting on makeup, or shaving—or, pain may occur spontaneously. Depending on the branch of the nerve that is affected, pain may also be triggered by brushing the teeth, eating, talking, or exposure to wind on the face. Fortunately, people rarely suffer from pain at night, and the pain does not usually disrupt sleep.

DIAGNOSIS

There is no definitive test for TN and diagnose is usually based on a patient's medical history, description of symptoms, physical exam, and a thorough neurological exam. Because of the large number of conditions that can cause facial pain, obtaining a correct diagnosis can be difficult, but finding the cause of the pain is important to appropriate treatment. Imaging with MRI or MRA may help to rule out a brain tumor or neurological illness such as MS.

TREATMENT

Treatment options include medicines, surgery, and complementary approaches. Antiseizure medications are often effective in helping to block nerve impulses and managing the pain of TN. These can include the following:

- carbamazepine
- oxcarbazepine
- topiramate
- clonazepam
- phenytoin
- lamotrigin
- gabapentin
- valproic acid

Tricyclic antidepressants such as amitriptyline or nortriptyline may be used to treat constant, burning, or aching pain. OTC analgesics and opioids are not usually helpful in treating the sharp, recurring pain caused by TN. If medications are tried but don't work, one of several neurosurgical procedures may be recommended. Unfortunately, some facial numbness may result after most of these surgical procedures, and it is possible for TN to reoccur at some point following surgery. Other possible risks of surgery include hearing loss, balance problems, infection, and stroke, so this possibility must be considered very carefully.

Effective CAM treatments for TN include injections of B-complex vitamins, a whole foods antiinflammatory diet, and acupuncture. For some people, avoiding chocolate and coffee seems to help prevent attacks.

Further information on TN can be obtained from the two organizations listed below, and from the National Institute of Neurolgical Disorders and Stroke, from which much of this information was drawn.

- American Chronic Pain Association. P.O. Box 850, Rocklin, CA 95677-0850. (916) 632-0922. http://members.tripod.com/<widdy/ACPA.html

- Trigeminal Neuralgia/Tic Douloureux Association. P.O. Box 340, Barnegat Light, NJ 08006. (609) 361-1014.

The next section of the book delves into the many possible causes of secondary headaches. Secondary headaches are far less common than the primary headache types already discussed, but they can be very serious, even life-threatening, as you'll see in the very next chapter.

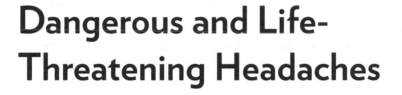

Dangerous and Life-Threatening Headaches

My day started out with my typical 3-mile morning run, but I didn't feel 100%. Something was off, so I returned home only half-way through my usual route. In the shower, I could feel a severe headache developing, and when I bent over to pick up the soap that slipped through my hands, I nearly passed out. I got out of the shower as quickly as I could, dried off and crawled back into bed. My wife was getting ready for work, and asked me if anything was wrong. I said that I had suddenly gotten an excruciating headache and almost fainted in the shower. I asked her to get me some ibuprofen and a glass of water. In the minute or so that she was gone, my world suddenly receded into blackness and I don't remember much else. When my wife returned, she had difficulty rousing me, I wasn't making sense, and my speech was slurred. She immediately called 911. Thankfully, they got me in right away, and there happened to be a neurologist on duty in the hospital that day. Imaging showed that I had a bleeding aneurysm. It hadn't catastrophically ruptured, which saved my life, but I still had to undergo emergency surgery—a craniotomy—to repair the defect in my blood vessel. And after that, I still wasn't out of the woods. My bleeding aneurysm had deprived parts of my brain of its critical blood supply, and I had to undergo months of therapy before I was able to regain enough of my previous function to resume normal life and return to my teaching job. I thank God that I wasn't alone when it happened, that I was able to get help right away, and that I have been able to recover nearly completely. JAMIE

Secondary headaches can have a multitude of causes. I'll focus on some of the most common, such as sinus infections, inflammatory autoimmune disorders, and mild head trauma, but I'll begin by providing important, possibly life-saving, information you need to know to recognize a "dangerous" headache.

When is a headache not just a headache? Anyone with a severe primary headache could tell you "It's not just a headache." But patients suffering from a secondary headache due to an underlying illness or condition need to be aware that some severe headache symptoms can be precursors or symptoms of a potentially life-threatening event. I've placed the most urgent and life-threatening of these conditions—strokes, aneurysms, and bleeding in the brain—in the beginning of these chapters on secondary headaches, followed by a discussion of another life-threatening disorder, bacterial meningitis.

Cerebrovascular Accident or Ischemic Stroke

The term stroke refers to a "cerebrovascular accident" (CVA), in which the brain is deprived of oxygen and nutrients when its normal blood supply is interrupted. What most people think of as a stroke is caused by a blood clot entering the cerebral circulation. The clot (or clots) occludes an artery in the brain, cutting off circulation to, and injuring, a specific area of brain tissue, which then begins to die. This results in loss of the function controlled by that area of the brain. A stroke can impair movement, sensation, communication, emotional stability, swallowing ability, and even vital functions like breathing, in which case the stroke is usually fatal.

Strokes come in all shapes and sizes, and they can have warning signs, known as "mini-strokes," or transient ischemic attacks (TIAs)—caused by a temporary disruption in blood flow through the brain. About 90% of all strokes are "ischemic strokes," caused by a blockage. One type of ischemic stroke, "thrombotic," occurs when a clot forms in the brain or the carotid arteries, often in an area narrowed by fatty deposits known as atherosclerosis. An "embolic" form of ischemic stroke occurs when a clot forms elsewhere in the body, and then travels through the bloodstream to the brain. Clots like these can form in the heart, especially in patients with atrial fibrillation—a weak, abnormal heart rhythm that prevents complete emptying of the chambers of the heart, allowing blood to pool and coagulate. For this reason, medications used to help treat atrial fibrillation also help to reduce the risk of stroke.

Risk factors for ischemic stroke include:

- Personal or family history
- Age greater than 55
- High blood pressure
- Diabetes
- High cholesterol
- Cigarette smoking
- Obesity
- Sedentary lifestyle
- Cardiovascular disease
- Abnormal heart rhythm—such as atrial fibrillation
- Use of contraceptive medications (even in young women)
- Binge drinking
- Use of the illicit heavy-duty drugs cocaine and methamphetamines

SYMPTOMS

Symptoms of stroke can come on suddenly and are often neurological in nature—involving some loss of function. Watch for these important signs and take immediate action to get help:

- *Sudden, severe headache,* possibly accompanied by vomiting, dizziness, or loss of consciousness.

- Sudden loss of balance/coordination, sudden dizziness, and difficulty walking.
- Sudden confusion, difficulty finding the appropriate word in a sentence, or incorrectly identifying an object. Slurred speech, sounding as if someone had too much to drink, is also common.
- Weakness, numbness, or paralysis on one side of the body. This may be as subtle as the inability to raise one eyebrow or a smile that droops at one end, or as severe as the inability to move both limbs on one side.
- Sudden blurred vision, double vision, or loss of sight in one or both eyes.

DIAGNOSIS

Diagnosis must be made quickly in an emergency medical setting. The physician will do a brisk but thorough physical/neurological exam, including checking the blood vessels at the back of the eyes with an ophthalmoscope. The patient will be asked questions about personal and family history, and vital signs will be assessed. Blood tests can identify problems with clotting and measure the level of blood glucose and other critical blood chemicals. Diagnostic imaging may be used to identify the area of stroke, or locate any active bleeding in the brain, to distinguish between ischemic and hemorrhage stroke, which are treated differently. CT plays a key role, but MRI, carotid ultrasound, or arteriography of the cerebral arteries may be used as well. The complete diagnostic workup may also include echocardiography to visualize the heart as it is beating, identifying factors that might have led to clot formation.

What Nurses Know...

If you notice these signs in someone you are with, even if they seem to come and go, call 911 or your local emergency services immediately. With strokes, every minute counts. The longer that brain cells continue to be deprived of oxygen, the greater the potential for cell death and brain damage.

TREATMENT

Until emergency services arrive, continue to observe the affected person and try to keep them calm. Be prepared to administer cardiopulmonary resuscitation rescue breaths if the person stops breathing. Administering oxygen by nasal cannula, if available, is another intervention to help oxygenate the brain.

If a stroke is identified as ischemic in origin, the patient may be given medications such as aspirin or other blood-thinning drugs like Coumadin (warfarin), heparin, or Plavix (clopidogrel). Ischemic strokes can also be treated quickly restore blood flow to the brain by using the "clot-busting" drug "tissue plasminogen activator" (TPA) intravenously within a short time, and at least within a 4-hour window following stroke. More invasive treatments include surgery to mechanically remove the occluding blood clot. Fortunately, stroke treatment has improved dramatically in the past decade and if initiated quickly after the initial symptoms, the chance of recovery is good for many patients. Follow-up treatment is then focused on preventing another stroke, through modifying lifestyle factors, taking specific medications, and sometimes undergoing preventive procedures.

PREVENTION

Ischemic stroke cannot always be prevented—there are some underlying medical conditions and genetic factors which increase the risk of stroke. But for many people, the risk of stroke can be greatly reduced by simply living a healthy lifestyle. Unfortunately, things seem to be moving in the wrong direction when it comes to reducing the rate of stroke. Ischemic strokes have been declining among seniors in the past decade or so, but they have been *increasing* among younger people. A recent Centers for Disease Control study compared numbers of strokes among various age groups between the years 1995 to 1996 and 2007 to 2008. The results were startling: In men ages 15 to 34, incidence of ischemic stroke increased 46%; women in this age bracket had a 23% increase. Sadly, many of these strokes were preventable. In the patients studied, risk factors were common and included high blood pressure; diabetes; poor cholesterol profile; obesity; and the abuse of tobacco, alcohol, and drugs. These are all, to large extent, modifiable risk factors. By eating a healthy diet, exercising, and maintaining a healthy weight, as well as by avoiding the use of tobacco, alcohol, and drugs, we can lower our risk for ischemic stroke.

Help is available from a variety of sources in your community. Insurance covers some preventive health programs so check with your health care provider about strategies to lower your risk of stroke.

Aneurysm and Brain Hemorrhage/Hemorrhagic Stroke

"Hemorrhagic strokes" occur due to the leaking or rupture of vessels in the brain, allowing blood to escape and damage brain tissue. Uncontrolled high-blood pressure can weaken the walls of blood vessels in the brain, leading to the development of aneurysms, or bulging balloon-like pouches in the blood vessel. Aneurysms can also be the result of congenital abnormalities of the blood vessels. There are two types of hemorrhagic strokes: those that occur within the brain, and those that occur just outside it, between the brain and the skull.

An estimated one in 15 people in the United States will develop a brain aneurysm during their lifetime, or in 8 to 10 million Americans. But it is likely that many people who do have aneurysms are not aware, and may remain unaware, unless symptoms develop. Unfortunately, these can sometimes happen abruptly and catastrophically when an aneurysm ruptures, which happens to about one in 100 people with aneurysms: Each year, roughly 30,000 people in the United States experience bleeding into the brain or the space between the brain and the brain's covering in the brain, as the result of a ruptured aneurysm. Startlingly, 10 to 15% of them will die before reaching the hospital. Nearly half will die within the following 30 days, while many patients who survive are left with permanent neurological impairment, including problems with memory, perception, and ability to carry out daily activities. Those in middle age, from 35 to 60, are most at risk, and women are more likely to suffer a brain aneurysm than men, by a ratio of 3:2.

Interrupting the blood supply to brain tissue can lead to the catastrophic outcomes associated with hemorrhagic stroke: brain damage or death. Aneurysms can be located anywhere in the brain but most often are found in an area at the base of the brain where the large arteries of the brain connect. Cerebral aneurysms can result from a congenital abnormality of an artery wall, or from an arteriovenous malformation (AVM), a tangle of arteries and veins in the brain that leads to circulatory problems and heightens the risk of rupture. People with vascular diseases or connective tissue disorders, those with a family history of aneurysm, those with high blood pressure, people with a history of head trauma, those of African American descent, and older people are at increased risk of developing a brain aneurysm.

Risk factors for rupture include having larger aneurysms (over 10 mm). In addition, there are several lifestyle factors, easily modified, which greatly increase the risk of suffering a ruptured cerebral aneurysm. These include heavy smoking, binge drinking, and cocaine use.

SYMPTOMS

Not all aneurysms rupture. Some may leak a small amount of blood into surrounding tissues, and some may grow large enough to create pressure on surrounding nerves or areas of the brain. When an aneurysm is very small and does not bleed, it often does not cause problems for patients; it may not even be discovered except through a random MRI ordered for other reasons. When the aneurysm enlarges, though, it may cause pain and a range of neurological symptoms affecting one side of the body, including: numbness, weakness or paralysis, a dilated pupil, visual field cuts which block or cut off part of the normal expanse of vision, difficulty moving one eye in all directions—for example, it may be difficult to look up or sideways—pain in the brow region, behind the eye, in the back of the skull, or in the upper neck.

Other symptoms of an enlarging, unruptured aneurysm include severe headache, blurred vision, sensitivity to light, and speech changes, depending on the area of the brain affected. These symptoms may develop gradually over time, leading patients to seek medical care. If neurological workup and imaging are able to identify an aneurysm, this allows an opportunity for possible life-saving treatments.

The first symptom of a ruptured brain aneurysm is commonly a sudden, severe headache, sometimes accompanied by nausea and vomiting, drooping eyelid, and behavior changes, including loss of consciousness. About half of people who suffer ruptured aneurysms report suffering a warning, or "sentinel headache" in the 2 weeks prior to rupture. But symptoms of a ruptured cerebral aneurysm often strike suddenly, without warning. Until you are evaluated by a physician, and in some cases, a neurologist, do not assume that the symptoms you are experiencing will pass, or that they can be self-treated! In some cases, taking certain medications could potentially be harmful to your condition. It is extremely important to seek emergency care if you have any of these signs and symptoms:

- Loss of consciousness or seizure. Seizure occurs in about 25% of patients with ruptured aneurysm.
- Any *very severe sudden headache which strikes without warning.*
- Acute confusion and altered mental status. It is immediately clear that something is suddenly wrong with the person.
- Any headache accompanied by fever, muscle soreness, nausea, or vomiting, a stiff neck, numbness, tingling or paralysis, or difficulty speaking.
- Any headache that develops following a head injury, even if you suspect it was just a minor fall or bump, especially if it worsens gradually. This is especially important if you take a blood-thinning medication, which can increase the risk of bleeding in the brain or surrounding areas.
- *Any sudden headache that you feel is the worst headache you've ever experienced,* or different than any headache you've ever experienced.

Other possibly serious signs that a headache should be investigated promptly include any headache that worsens over several days and/or changes in pattern, any new headache that develops over age 50, and any headache that routinely occurs upon sneezing, coughing, or bending over.

DIAGNOSIS

Many aneurysms remain undiscovered or are discovered when people are being evaluated or treated for another condition. But if your doctor does suspect a brain aneurysm, based on any of the symptoms listed previously, you may be asked to undergo the following tests:

- A CT scan, or a computed tomography angiogram (CTA), which is better at evaluating blood vessels than standard CT, can help to locate bleeding in the brain.
- A lumbar puncture to look for blood in your cerebrospinal fluid (CSF) helps to identify subarachnoid hemorrhage.
- Magnetic resonance angiography (MRA) is similar to CTA but uses a magnetic field in combination with pulsed radio waves to create precise pictures of blood vessels in the brain.
- A cerebral angiogram involves injecting dye into the cerebral artery and allows the aneurysm to be seen on x-ray. Although this test is more invasive and carries greater risk, it allows the radiologist to locate brain aneurysms smaller than 5 mm.

In the event of ruptured aneurysm and hemorrhage, these tests may take the place of a routine neurological exam, which would take too long in an emergency situation. According to family or other witnesses, it is usually clear that something is catastrophically wrong, and urgent action is required. If symptoms are more subtle, a thorough neurological and physical exam is indicated.

Early diagnosis and treatment are very important when dealing with aneurysms and may lead to more successful outcomes. Treatment for an unruptured aneurysm involves little recovery time, while recovery after rupture may take weeks to months of rehabilitation. But most people with aneurysms are not aware of it, and unfortunately sometimes find out in a catastrophic event.

TREATMENT

Hemorrhage from a ruptured aneurysm requires immediate life-saving treatment to stop the bleeding in the brain and prevent permanent damage. In some cases, surgery is needed to remove large amounts of blood in order to relieve pressure on the brain. This emergency treatment is followed by bed rest and supportive care and rehabilitation. A secondary but extremely important goal is to repair the defect to prevent a recurrence, which happens in 20% to 30% of patients who have had one aneurysm.

Several techniques are used for unruptured aneurysms: the older but still-utilized "surgical clipping," and the newer "coil embolization." There is also the option of continuing to observe, while avoiding surgery. This option is usually confined to small, non-bleeding aneurysms, in which the risk of rupture is low and does not outweigh the considerable risks of brain surgery. These patients may be closely followed to monitor growth in the aneurysm, to track symptoms, and treat risk factors such as hypertension (high blood pressure). Neurosurgeons also weigh such risks as age, cardio-vascular status, and overall health before deciding on a treatment approach.

Surgical clipping is done to decrease the pressure on the aneurysm and reduce the risk of rupture. The surgeon places a small metal clip around the base of the aneurysm, which isolates it from normal blood circulation. Not all aneurysms are suitable for this procedure, and require complete dissection. In these cases the cut ends of the blood vessels are stitched together, or rarely, a donor vessel must be inserted.

In coil embolization, a small surgical tube is placed into the affected artery near the weakened blood vessel. Tiny metal coils resembling a small spring are moved through the tube into the aneurysm, helping to stabilize the weakened blood vessel walls, while also helping to block off the blood vessel. This less-invasive procedure also reduces the risk of rupture, and is believed to be safer than surgical clipping. A patient undergoing these procedures will be hospitalized in intensive care for close monitoring.

Bleeding in the Brain

Older adults may be at higher risk of bleeding in the brain, which can result in a subdural hematoma or other medical emergency often related to falls. All falls in older adults and in persons taking blood thinners should be reported to a physician, especially when the head strikes the ground or a hard object.

SYMPTOMS

Sometimes injuries cause a slow bleeding of vessels in the brain and are not noticed immediately. Continued tracking may be necessary for several weeks in some situations. Bleeding, or hemorrhage, in the brain is an important and dangerous complication of head trauma. There are three main categories:

- A subarachnoid hemorrhage is the term for active bleeding beneath the arachnoid layer (or between the arachnoid layer and the pia mater, which lies closest to the brain) that occurs as a result of trauma, or more rarely, occurs spontaneously from the rupture of a cerebral aneurysm. Sudden, severe headache is the most common symptom of subarachnoid hemorrhage, and patients who have survived describe it as "the worst headache they have ever experienced." Nausea, vomiting, neck pain and stiffness, drowsiness, confusion, and sensitivity to light are common. If symptoms come on more gradually, neurological symptoms including arm and leg numbness or weakness usually affecting one side of the body, difficulty speaking and swallowing, and facial weakness (including one-sided facial droop) may occur. If symptoms progress, the patient can develop seizures, lose consciousness, and fall into a coma. Subarachnoid hemorrhage is a medical emergency and it is necessary to act quickly.
- A subdural hematoma is a collection of blood in the thin space between the arachnoid layer and the dura mater. Blood pooling in this area can be the result of tearing of the blood vessels in these tissues during a head trauma. Symptoms can include: confusion, disorientation, headache, problems with sensation and lack of coordination, vision changes, behavior or demeanor changes, difficulty speaking, seizures, vomiting, and loss of consciousness. A subdural hematoma can be chronic or acute and is considered a medical emergency.
- An epidural hematoma is a similar collection of blood in the cranial epidural space, between the dura and the bone of the skull. This accumulation of blood can occur as a result of accident, injury, or occasionally occurs spontaneously, and it is found in up to 15% of fatal head injuries. In fact, epidural hematoma is considered the most serious complication related to traumatic head injury, and is always a medical emergency. Symptoms can include: severe headache, nausea, vomiting, seizures, and neurological symptoms such as vision changes, difficulty speaking, weakness, and numbness.

DIAGNOSIS AND TREATMENT

Diagnosis is made based on the radiologist's reading of the CT scan of the brain, which is good at showing doctors where the acute bleeding is occurring. Treatments depend on the size of the hematoma and the condition of the patient. Surgery may be necessary to stop ongoing bleeding. Recovery time following craniotomy, or surgery within the head, is also variable, but with appropriate therapies complete recovery is possible for many patients.

Bacterial Meningitis

Meningitis is an infection of the meninges, the multilayer protective covering of the brain and spinal cord. Bacterial meningitis is serious and can be fatal due to its effects of severe and often prolonged inflammation surrounding the brain and spinal cord—and this condition is considered to be a medical emergency. This is why an early goal of diagnosis is to determine whether the condition is "viral" or "bacterial." Bacterial meningitis occurs only in about 3 per 100,000 individuals annually in developed countries like the United States. Viral meningitis is more than three times as common, and it can also cause serious discomfort. But viral meningitis is considered to be less serious than bacterial meningitis, which if left untreated, is nearly always fatal. This discussion will focus on bacterial meningitis.

In adults, more than three-quarters of meningitis cases are caused by two pathogens: *Neisseria meningitides* and *Streptococcus pneumoniae.* In bacterial meningitis, bacteria are carried to the meninges through general circulation, or they come into direct contact with the meninges via the nasal and sinus cavities. Head trauma involving skull fracture is a significant risk factor for meningitis, since this allows bacteria from the nasal cavity to come into contact with the meningeal membranes. Rarely, an infection in the head or neck can lead to meningitis.

SYMPTOMS

The patient with meningitis looks and feels and very ill—with fever, pounding headache, and pronounced stiffness in the neck. Neck stiffness is often less evident in very young children, who may instead show behavior changes such as refusal to take in nourishment, increased irritability, and drowsiness. Infants under 6 months of age with meningitis may show a bulging fontanelle—the soft spot at the top of the head where the plates of the skull have not yet fused together. Older children, teens, and adults may show symptoms such as confusion, vomiting, and extreme sensitivity to light and sound. But the most common symptom of meningitis is severe headache affecting both sides of the head, which may develop before the onset of neck rigidity—an inability to flex the neck forward (with the chin toward the chest) more than a few inches.

DIAGNOSIS

Early recognition and treatment are the keys to preventing fatal complications. For accurate diagnosis of the patient with meningitis symptoms it is often necessary to perform a lumbar puncture to obtain a sample of cerebrospinal fluid (CSF)—the clear, watery, substance that surrounds and cushions the brain and spinal cord. Also known as a "spinal tap," this procedure involves needle aspiration of CSF from the spinal canal. A local anesthetic is used and the somewhat uncomfortable procedure takes only a few minutes. A lumbar puncture can provide critical information that will lead to successful treatment and recovery. The CSF sample is tested for the presence and type of white blood cells, red blood cells, protein content, glucose level, and bacteria—including techniques to identify the specific microorganism causing the infection.

Your doctor will also perform a complete neurological exam, including tests exclusive to meningitis which may include asking the patient to bend the knees or shake the head rapidly side-to-side. The skin over the body, arms, and legs will be examined for the presence of a rash—a sign that the meningitis may be caused by meningococcal bacteria. The rash associated with "meningococcal meningitis" consists of multiple small purplish spots covering the body, extremities, and/or mucous membranes, and it may precede other symptoms such as headache.

TREATMENT

Bacterial meningitis is a life-threatening disease that requires hospitalization and treatment with strong antibiotics directed at the bacteria causing the illness, supportive care of the patient with IV fluids, and attentive nursing care. People with seizures are treated with anticonvulsants. Some critically-ill patients may temporary need assistance with breathing. In meningitis, the brain tissue may swell, leading to decreased level of consciousness with abnormalities in body posture and pupillary reflexes. In some situations, the use of corticosteroids may be used to prevent serious complications related to brain swelling. Long-term consequences of meningitis can include loss of hearing, visual symptoms, seizure disorders, and mental retardation—especially when this disease occurs in infants and toddlers.

PREVENTION

Both bacterial and viral meningitis are contagious and can be spread through respiratory secretions and "close contact": Kissing, sneezing, and coughing are common means of transmission. In the years before antibiotics and vaccines, meningitis was often fatal. Now we have powerful tools to help prevent serious complications and death. There are also now preventive vaccines available for meningococci, pneumococci, and *Haemophilus influenzae* type B. Speak with your doctor about getting these vaccines.

Brain Tumor, Pseudotumor, and Acoustic Neuroma

A severe, persistent headache accompanied by neurological symptoms can be scary, and it can even make patients think the worst—that they have a life-threatening brain tumor. Brain tumors are rarely the cause of such a headache, but knowing how to recognize when you need help for a serious medical condition is critically important. I'll discuss three conditions with similar symptoms.

Brain Tumor: Who Gets Them and Why?

Only about one in 29,000 men and one in 38,000 women will develop a brain tumor each year. People living in industrialized countries have roughly twice the risk of suffering a brain tumor as those in underdeveloped nations. Dr. Christina Peterson, a

What Nurses Know…

Patients with either the viral or bacterial form of meningitis often suffer severe pain, weakness, and nausea. They may want to curl up in a ball and be left alone, but this puts them at risk of serious dehydration and does not allow regular nursing assessment of a patient's medical status. Sensitivity to sound is nearly always present, and sensitivity to light can be extreme. They may insist on keeping the drapes or shades drawn and the lights out in the room at all times, which of course makes it very hard to provide care. Encourage the patient to take fluids, make every effort to maintain a quiet environment, and offer the person ear plugs. Try using the lowest setting on lights, and turn lights off when you leave the room. Provide dark sunglasses for the person to wear when the lights do need to be on, however briefly.

headache specialist in Portland, Oregon, writes reassuringly about headaches in brain tumor. "Although up to 70% of people with various brain tumors have a headache at the time of diagnosis, only about 8% of tumor patients have headache as their first and only symptom."

SYMPTOMS

Although some sources describe the headache of brain tumor as a "dull pain," there is great variability and no "typical brain tumor headache." Sometimes brain tumors can occur *without* associated headache pain. Brain tumor headaches are different than headache symptoms in other headache disorders such as migraine, according to some patients who have experienced both. Unfortunately, the symptoms of a brain tumor often develop gradually and may be mild and nonspecific. In some cases, a neurological disorder or even an infection can cause symptoms that may *mimic* a brain tumor. But there are some clues that doctors look for in order to rule out a tumor, or neoplasm, when patients complain of headache:

- Headaches that are worse in the morning and lessen throughout the day.
- New headache in a patient over age fifty without a previous headache history.
- Headache brought on by bending over or shaking the head vigorously.
- Headache limited to a very specific area of the head and no other location. Even then the chances of a brain tumor are still low. If headache location changes it is very unlikely to be related to a brain tumor.
- A headache accompanied by "focal" neurologic signs. "Focal" means a specific nerve pathway or area of the brain is affected—one which controls a specific function or is associated with a specific location such as the left side of the face, problems with speech, or an area with limited sensation.
- A headache accompanied by signs of increased intracranial pressure—or pressure within the skull which affects the brain and CSF. These include: vomiting without accompanying nausea, swelling of the head of the optic nerve, visual disturbances, loss of vision, and decreased level of consciousness. Additional signs include increased systolic blood pressure, slowed heart rate, and irregular breathing. Increased intracranial pressure has a high likelihood of injuring brain tissue, especially if it is prolonged. Following head trauma, for example, one of the goals of emergency treatment is to attempt to relieve or reduce intracranial pressure.
- A headache accompanied or followed by the development of new onset seizures. Seizures are a common complication of brain tumors. They can be generalized "grand mal" seizures or more subtle "focal" seizures involving only one part of the body.

DIAGNOSIS

Ideally, a neurooncologist—a doctor with special training in studying cancer and neurology—will coordinate the diagnostic workup of a patient with signs or symptoms suggestive of a brain tumor. Imaging studies of the brain will be ordered to identify the brain

What Nurses Know...

A primary malignant tumor at a distant site in the body may produce cells that break away from the main tumor and travel through the circulation to the brain, where these cells produce secondary or "metastatic" tumors. Metastatic brain tumors are the most common type of brain tumor seen by neurosurgeons, and in adults, lung cancer is the most common primary source of brain metastases. Other cancers that may lead to metastatic brain tumors include breast, kidney, and colon, but a great many brain tumors arise directly from tissues within the brain.

tumor location and size, while other imaging studies of the chest, abdomen, and pelvis may be ordered to attempt to locate the primary tumor, which usually also requires surgery or other treatment. Imaging studies may include an MRI and especially a CT, which is very good at showing doctors areas of bleeding or fluid build-up within the brain. A PET scan may be ordered in some situations. If imaging scans raise no red flags but a patient's symptoms are suspicious, a spinal tap may be done to obtain a sample of CSF to examine for the presence of cancer cells.

TREATMENT

The type of treatment depends on the type of cancer involved, the location of the tumor or tumors, and other specifics. Steroid medications may be given to immediately reduce swelling in the brain, which helps to alleviate symptoms. Treating patients effectively for pain is often necessary as well. Single or isolated tumors may be surgically removed. Chemotherapy may be ordered, and the patient may undergo targeted radiation using precisely-focused radio-surgical techniques.

PSEUDOTUMOR CEREBRI OR FALSE BRAIN TUMOR

Pseudotumor cerebri, also called "idiopathic intracranial hypertension" or "false brain tumor," is a condition in which symptoms mimic those of brain tumor. This condition can occur in various age groups but is most common in women of child-bearing age, and obesity is a very significant risk-factor. Pseudotumor cerebri occurs in only one in 100,000 people, but obese women under age 44 have nearly 20 times the risk of developing this disorder. Unfortunately, untreated pseudotumor cerebri carries a high risk of causing permanent vision loss due to chronic swelling surrounding the optic nerve. Blindness eventually results in as many as 10% of patients. Symptoms overlap with those of brain tumor, and may include:

- Headache behind the eyes severe enough to wake patients from sleep.
- Headaches that seem to be worsened by moving the eyes.
- Ringing in the ears coordinating with the pulse.
- Nausea and vomiting, sometimes accompanied by dizziness.
- Vision changes, including blurry, darkened, or double vision; loss of peripheral vision; seeing flashes of light, or transient loss of vision in one or both eyes.

Symptoms may be worsened if you hold your breath and tighten your abdominal muscles, as sometimes happens when straining to have a bowel movement. Some patients may also have pain in the upper body affecting the neck and shoulders.

Excess CSF is responsible for causing pseudotumor; this may be due to a problem with absorption into the bloodstream, or a narrowing in the opening to two large cavities beneath the brain which allow blood to drain from the back of the head. In addition, there may be a connection between this disorder and the endocrine system, in particular the adrenal glands or the parathyroid glands.

Diagnosis involves checking the eye for characteristic swelling in the optic disk and testing the patient's vision to help identify blind spots.

Treatment is focused on controlling the symptoms and protecting the patient's vision. If you are overweight, you will be encouraged to lose weight. Surgery may be necessary to reduce the pressure surrounding the optic nerve and this can be done using a small, thin, flexible tube called an endoscope. Medications used to treat Pseudotumor cerebri include the glaucoma drug Diamox (acetazolamide), along with the diuretic Lasix (furosemide), and typical migraine medications to address the severe headache. If the condition persists, surgeons can implant a tube in the brain to drain excess CSF into the abdomen. This is called a ventriculoperitoneal (VP) shunt. This procedure improves symptoms for more than 80% of patients, but carries with it the risk of infection.

ACOUSTIC NEUROMA

Acoustic Neuroma (AN), also called auditory tumor, occurs in less than one per 100,000 people, although diagnosis is rising as a result of improved imaging techniques. This "benign" tumor develops in the tissue of the nerve that connects the inner ear to the brain. It is located deep inside the back of the inner ear canal just under the brain, and it grows at a very slow pace.

The primary symptom of AN is hearing loss on one side, but headache is also present in about half of patients at the time they are diagnosed. Headaches, balance problems and/or dizziness, may increase with tumor size. Patients may complain of feeling a heaviness in the head and neck, which is worse in the morning and at night, which is aggravated by position changes, coughing, or sneezing. Gradual hearing loss may be due to injury. Sudden or fluctuating hearing loss, which affects a smaller percentage of patients, may be due to disruption of the cochlear blood supply. Tinnitus, or ringing in the ear, facial numbness, and vertigo are less common symptoms of AN.

Doctors who specialize in diagnosing and treating ear, nose, and throat disorders are called otorhinolaryngologists. These specialists, along with neurologists and hearing specialists may be involved in the diagnosis and treatment of AN. Patient history and physical examination will be followed by a series of tests to evaluate hearing and balance, two important functions controlled by the eighth cranial nerve. CT and MRI are useful in identifying tumor location and size.

What Nurses Know...

A benign tumor is not "cancerous." It does not spread to other parts of the body and rarely grows back when surgically removed. Benign tumors can still cause damage by growing large enough to press on vital organs or tissues, a problem that is more dangerous if the tumor is in a confined space like the skull.

Microsurgery of various types is still the treatment of choice for AN, but older patients with small tumors may be able to avoid surgery if followed carefully by their doctors. Treatment may also focus on slowing or stopping tumor growth by using a special type of low-dose radiation targeted to a very precise point using a special device, while minimizing the potential harm to surrounding tissues that can occur with more widespread radiation.

Recognizing the symptoms of AN early and seeking appropriate treatment helps to increase the chances of complete recovery. But there are significant risks inherent in any intra-cranial surgery, including AN removal surgery. These can include permanent hearing and vision loss, and possibly facial paralysis. So, patients who have the misfortune to develop a tumor on the same side as their only seeing eye or only hearing ear are of special concern and they may decide to forego surgery. But one of the most common and debilitating possible complications is *severe, chronic postoperative headache.*

Many patients report persistent headaches following AN surgery. The Acoustic Neuroma Association (ANA) completed a survey of more than 1,600 patients in 2005, which has helped to clarify the significance of postoperative headaches. Half of those who responded reported having headaches more than once a day, lasting from 1 to 4 hours, with most patients rating their headaches as moderate-to-severe. In studies, postoperative headaches were more common in women and were reported to be more intense than in men. Younger patients tended to also rate their headaches as more severe than older patients. Patients who reported frequent headaches before AN surgery were more likely to also experience more daily headaches after surgery. Postoperative headache is usually treated with analgesics, and if severe, with a controlled course of narcotics. Patients with persistent or severe headaches may be referred to a chronic pain specialist.

Healing does reduce the occurrence of daily or near daily postoperative headaches and many patients reported that they stopped having headaches within about 3 months. Slightly more than a third, though, continue to have postoperative headaches, but even these longer-lasting headaches usually resolve within 3 years. But 3 years can seem like a very long time to a chronic headache patient.

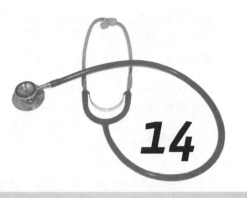

Headaches Related to Head Injury

Sometimes it seems that becoming a mother of boys (MOB) means learning to live with fear! From rock climbing, to downhill ski racing, mountain biking, and jumping off cliffs, to the new sport of parkour (free-running), there seems to be a risk of head injury lurking around every corner. My three-year old son suffered a fall from a fire truck to a concrete floor during a preschool field trip. He suffered a short loss of consciousness and did not speak for the first few hours after the fall. Fortunately, a CAT scan revealed no serious injury. From the height of the fall onto a concrete floor and his small size, we were all worried about a skull fracture. We simply observed him for neurological signs, nausea, vomiting, or excessive drowsiness. Sometimes being a nurse comes in handy.   WENDY

Millions of people suffer head injuries each year. Almost half of these come from auto accidents, and another 30% from fall, which are particularly common in children and seniors. Head injuries may also be the result of work-related accidents, hard hits from football or boxing, and violent assaults. Since head injuries are so common, it's fortunate that many victims will experience head pain for only a few days following injury. Unfortunately, about a third of people with head injuries may continue to suffer from headaches for several months, or longer, as part of an overall condition known as traumatic brain injury (TBI). This is also known as postconcussion syndrome. I'll use the term PCS for consistency.

Postconcussion Syndrome and Posttraumatic Headache

What is PCS? The delicate brain tissue can take a long time to heal, and while healing is taking place, or if the brain sustains an injury that cannot heal, patients experience many cognitive, behavioral, and psychological symptoms, as well as chronic headaches. In PCS, symptoms vary widely, and can include: changes in concentration and memory, communication problems (such as slurred speech), and changes in personality or behavior—including fatigue, apathy, irritability, and anger outbursts. Mood swings, depression, and loss of interest in life can vary from subtle effects, to significant problems that greatly impair one's ability to navigate work, family life, and social relationships. But, overall, headaches are an important clinical feature and are the most common symptom of PCS, occurring in up to 78% of patients following mild TBI. "Posttraumatic headache" (PTH) affects up to 450,000 people in the United States each year, often leaving patients with lingering symptoms. In this chapter, we'll learn how different types of head trauma can create chronic headaches and how these headaches can be treated. We'll take a look at three groups that are particularly vulnerable: children, athletes, and active-duty military personnel.

The Vulnerable Brain

Humans have hard heads. We are protected by the cranial bones of the skull, and the cranial meninges surrounding the much softer brain tissue. The three layers of meninges, the innermost pia mater, the arachnoid, and the outer dura mater, help to protect and cushion the brain, assisted by a layer of cerebrospinal fluid (CSF) circulating around and through the brain and throughout the contiguous spinal cord. Like all fluids, CSF is a built-in shock-absorber, helping to protect the delicate brain tissue from damage that could occur as the brain crashes against the inner surface of the bony skull. Both too little spinal fluid, caused by a CSF leak, and too much spinal fluid, caused by inadequate drainage, can quickly result in neurological changes and symptoms such as severe headache, severe nausea, and sensory disturbances.

Even with this superbly-designed protective system, head trauma can still occur, and the effects can last for months, years, or be permanent. Brain injuries due to head trauma usually result from the shuffling or bouncing of brain tissue against the hard surface of the bony skull, but they do not require a direct impact to the head. Shaken-baby syndrome is just one example of a TBI not caused by direct impact. Head injury also does not require a person to suffer a loss of consciousness, a common misconception.

When force is exerted against the head, causing a skull fracture, the fracturing of the skull bones helps to divert the force from reaching the brain. But when the skull does not fracture, the energy from the force cannot escape and is applied directly to the brain. This type of injury, called a contrecoup injury, can result in "axonal shearing"—causing damage to individual nerve cells in the brain. This disrupts communication between the neurons in the brain, causing various neurological effects.

There are a few other factors that increase the vulnerability of the brain to traumatic injury. The brain tissue is soft and somewhat flexible, and the brain itself is suspended on a stalk, which allows the head to move freely forward and back, or side to side, during an injury event—sometimes resulting in a "whiplash injury." This suspended position makes the brain particularly susceptible to side-blows that twist the brain stem, sending a flurry of overwhelming impulses to the brain, often causing unconsciousness—a "knock-out."

Skull fractures can tear the meninges and lead to leaking of the protective CFS, allowing bacteria to enter the brain cavity and possibly leading to life-threatening meningitis. Damage to the brain can also result from uncontrolled bleeding in, or around, the brain. The direct impact of head injuries on the brain is significant, but such injuries can be also release damaging free radicals, charged oxygen molecules which can harm tissues at the cellular level—the kind of damage that is harder to detect. And it's important to understand that even mild TBIs have additives effect equivalent to a more serious brain injury. We have seen this problem in sports-related injuries, child abuse, and war-related brain injuries, and new research has shown a connection between head injury earlier in life and two degenerative disorders: Alzheimer's disease and Parkinson's disease.

Types of Head Trauma

The three major types of brain injuries can be categorized as concussions, contusions, and lacerations, briefly described below.

CONCUSSION

The most common brain injury is a "concussion," which involves an abrupt, temporary loss of consciousness after an impact. This can be a result of a fall onto a hard surface, or as a result of a direct blow to the head. There is no visible bruising or bleeding of the brain but there may be some memory loss, especially for the period immediately preceding the injury. This temporary amnesia can have a peculiar specificity. I once had a head-injury patient who was struck by an auto while riding a bike. The patient's amnesia was personal—they did not remember their name. But, they did know the name of the company where they worked, its location, and even that they had gone out to get some lunch! The patient's coworkers were able to quickly able to make an identification by our description, and the accident victim very fortunately recovered completely within 24 hours.

Children may be particularly susceptible to head injury, and in fact, some doctors feel that TBI in children is underdiagnosed, instead attributed to behavioral or learning disorders. A new study, though, shows that hospitalizing children for observation isn't necessary for most children with minor head injuries, as long as there are no neurological problems and a head CT comes back clean. If children are able to eat and drink, and there are no signs of nausea or vomiting, taking them home and continuing to observe them closely may be best for children and their families. The same advice most likely applies to young, healthy adults with minor head injury, with one caveat: Adults with minor head injury should not drive, operate machinery, or take any medications without clearance from a physician.

CONTUSION

A "contusion" is a more serious head injury, causing a visible bruising to the brain. The brain's innermost protective covering, the pia mater, may be torn away over the area of injury, potentially allowing a blood clot to form in the subarachnoid space. Usually, with a contusion, there is a more extended loss of consciousness, lasting up to several hours.

LACERATION

A "laceration" involves a tearing of the brain tissue itself, from a severe skull fracture or a penetrating head wound such as a gunshot. The large blood vessels are ruptured and bleeding into the brain and subarachnoid space occur. This results in swelling and increased intracranial pressure, with associated neurological and physiological symptoms. Tearing of the brain tissue also increases the risk for cerebral hematoma, or a pooling of blood in a specific area, which may place pressure on the brain, and sometimes must be evacuated using surgical techniques.

The brain has an amazing capacity to heal, but there is some evidence that the ability to heal from TBI decreases with age, and with repeated injury, as we've learned when treating soldiers with PTH.

Posttraumatic Headache

As with other chronic headaches, chronic PTHs are most often tension-type headaches (75%), followed by migraine without aura (21%), and less frequently, migraine with aura. Some patients may experience occipital neuralgia as an aching feeling of pressure due to muscular entrapment of the greater occipital nerve, or as the result of referred pain from activated trigger points in the suboccipital, upper trapezius, or semi-spinalis capitis muscles. In occipital neu-ralgia, the back of the head feels sore when light pressure is applied, and firm pressure reproduces the typical headache.

In one study comparing characteristics of natural headaches with those of PTHs there were no obvious differences, leading researchers to conclude that they may be generated by similar processes.

SYMPTOMS

The headache resulting from mild-to-moderate head injuries begins almost immediately, and can include an aching, throbbing feeling of pain encompassing the entire head, or more localized sensations of stabbing pain or pressure. If an area of the head impacted a hard surface, there is often also quite noticeable swelling—the typi-cal "goose-egg." But "invisible" swelling can also be taking place inside the brain. The headache can be intense and debilitating. These types of headache are often worsened by any type of activity, and the patient is likely to seek rest. Drowsiness can also accom-pany head injury, but falling asleep if you are alone is not a good idea. Patients need to seek help. They will need someone to moni-tor their condition because later symptoms can include anxiety, impaired memory, dizziness, nausea, and vomiting, or even more serious symptoms like seizures. Even minor trauma to the head or neck can occasionally produce a pattern of severe chronic head-aches, including head injuries with minimal loss of consciousness, and headaches from whiplash.

DIAGNOSIS

Diagnosis of PTH is based on a history of injury, and complaints of headache and other associated symptoms. The ICHD-II criteria state that the onset of headache must occur less than 7 days after head injury to be classified as a "posttraumatic" headache. Chronic PTH requires that symptoms persist for more than 3 months. Diagnostic imaging helps to rule out bleeding in the brain, lesions, and skull fracture, but many patients with PTH show no special diagnostic findings. Newer, more sensitive imaging techniques may help to remedy this.

TREATMENT

Although it may take many months to obtain a diagnosis of PTH, treatment with prophylactic headache medications has shown positive results, at least in the case of posttraumatic migraine, with 70% of patients reporting significant improvement. Overall, the majority of patients with PTH can be treated successfully, achieving good headache control within 6 to 12 months. Prophylactic medications can include: beta blockers (usually propranolol), antidepressants, calcium channel blockers, monoamine oxidase inhibitors, and anticonvulsants. Drugs used to treat acute symptoms can include triptans and ergotamine derivatives, or, less frequently, controlled-release long-acting opiates.

More recently, occipital nerve blocks, including a local anesthetic and a corticosteroid, have provided patients short-term, and in some cases, even long-term relief. Unfortunately, up to 20% may continue to suffer from PTH for many years, or indefinitely. These patients often continue to have life-long problems with thinking, behavior and communication, as well as seizure disorders. Because of the psychological and cognitive aspects of PTH, an interdisciplinary or "holistic" approach is important. CAM treatments including physical therapy, biofeedback, myofascial trigger point release, and injection techniques have had some success in treating PTHs. Patients and families may benefit from ongoing counseling.

Posttraumatic Headache in Children

Head injuries can take place at home, in school, or when participating in athletics. Those who play high-impact sports such as football, hockey, rugby, and even soccer are at higher risk for a serious head injury—one that might produce a chronic PTH. Children have been injured by falling from horses and tree-houses, and from crashing while downhill skiing or riding a bicycle. Helmets help, and should always be worn when participating in these active sports. In fact, many experts feel that parents often underestimate the risks of a child suffering a head injury while riding a bike, scooter, or four-wheeler, and remind us that brain injury can result from falling as little as 2 feet!

PREVENTING TRAUMATIC BRAIN INJURY AND PCS

Among children, TBI is most common in those under five, and in adolescent males age 15 and older. The Centers for Disease Control (CDC) has issued the following safety tips:

- Wear a seatbelt every time you drive or ride in a car.
- Buckle your child into a child safety seat, booster seat, or seatbelt (depending on the child's age) every time the child rides in a car.
- Wear a helmet and make sure your children wear helmets when
  - riding a bike or motorcycle.
  - playing a contact sport such as football or ice hockey.
  - using in-line skates, riding a skateboard, or riding a scooter.
  - batting and running bases in baseball or softball.
  - riding a horse.
  - skiing or snowboarding.
- Keep firearms and bullets stored in a locked cabinet when not in use.
- Avoid falls by
  - using a step-stool with a grab-bar to reach objects on high shelves.
  - installing handrails on stairways.
  - installing window guards to keep young children from falling out of open windows.
  - using safety gates at the top and bottom of stairs when young children are around.
- Make sure the surface on your child's playground is made of shock-absorbing material (e.g., hardwood mulch, sand).

Posttraumatic Headache in Athletes

Amateur and professional sports are important sources of head injuries resulting in PCS and PTH. Many of you may be familiar with the tragic outcome of boxer Mohammed Ali's repeated blows to the head: parkinson's disease. But there are many other sports-related injuries that occur in prominent athletes each year, sometimes with career-ending effects. Could these injuries be prevented?

What Nurses Know...

WHEN TO SEEK HELP FOR YOUR CHILD

It is not always easy to tell how serious a head injury is, or whether it is likely to produce lingering effects, but there are some key signs and symptoms to be aware of, and which should prompt parents and caregivers to seek medical care immediately following a head injury.

Parents, caregivers, coaches, teachers, and others who are responsible for children need to be alert and observant, and seek help in these situations:

- *When a child complains of headache following a fall or a blow to the head, however minor it appeared.*
- *When pain is severe or accompanied by excessive drowsiness, dizziness, memory loss, nausea, vomiting, vision changes, neck pain or stiffness, changes in behavior such as confusion, problems with coordination and balance, or fever.*
- *When a child has clear, watery drainage from the nose after a head injury: This could be CSF, a sign that the protective membrane has been punctured, potentially allowing bacteria to enter the sterile space of the central nervous system, a potentially life-threatening situation.*
- *When you suspect seizure activity in a child: This needs to be observed and evaluated by a neurologist.*
- *When an infant or toddler exhibits persistent, inconsolable crying and refusal to nurse or drink from a bottle. They may be impossible to soothe with the usual comfort strategies.*

Baseball player Corey Koskie tumbled backward during a game in a fall that resulted in PCS. "My head hurt, my body was numb, I couldn't walk through a door, I couldn't go in the sun, I couldn't enjoy time with my kids, my stress level was through the roof, everybody was telling me I'm fine and I wasn't," Koskie explained to a sports reporter. And he noted that the "hidden" nature of head injuries makes it difficult for people to understand why athletes aren't soon back on the field, unlike with injuries that result in a cast or knee-brace. Although Koskie ultimately recovered enough to return to the sport he loves, the process required extensive physical therapy and took over 2½ years! Giants' catcher Mike Matheny wasn't so lucky—he was forced to retire early due to his PCS.

PCS injuries in baseball actually occur much less frequently than in high impact sports like football and ice hockey. In 2009, Tampa Bay Lightning goaltender Mike Smith was injured in a game, preventing him from playing professional hockey for several weeks during peak season. Boston Bruins' star Marc Savard has also suffered the consequences of PCS, keeping him out of the action and disappointing hockey fans. But, as Savard agreed in a *Boston Globe* interview, he has had lingering issues with nausea, headache, fatigue, dizziness, visual effects, memory loss, and depression. Savard also pointed out that head injuries differ dramatically from orthopedic injuries, and they need extra time to heal before resuming play. There has since been a call for a ban on hits to the head following several high-profile hockey-related head injuries.

Former Pittsburg Steeler Merril Hoge also knows first-hand how the high-impact sport of football might impact the brain. His bright career ended at the young age of 30, following a bad case of PCS, followed by a premature attempt to return to play. He now uses his own experience with PCS, including persistent headaches, neck pains, and vision problems, to educate youth football coaches about preventing head trauma. Hoge has said the in order to reduce the risk of head trauma in players, the "culture of football" has to change. These changes include teaching players that "leading with the head" is dangerous and that there is no such thing as a concussion-proof helmet. Hoge suggests that coaches work on helping young athletes strengthen core muscles that support the neck, and making sure that athletes' helmets fit properly. And he is adamant that all players should be removed from a game at the first sign of a head injury, and be evaluated thoroughly before they are cleared to return.

TREATMENT

The saying that "time heals all wounds" sadly does not apply to every case of PCS. Time is important, but in some cases, it is not enough. Medications are used, along with cognitive therapies to restore normal function. And there are some new developments in the treatment of PCS:

- Studies are looking at the effect of hyperbaric oxygen therapy, which may accelerate healing and speed recovery time.
- CAM therapies such as myofascial release and myofascial trigger point therapy may be of use with injuries involving the back of the head and neck, including some whiplash injuries.
- A new treatment for athletes with PCS is being pioneered at the University of Buffalo. Conventional advice for recovering from PCS has been to have the patient avoid exertion and to rest. But some studies have shown that patients who rested for significant periods of time following PCS, as part of their overall treatment plan, did not recover any faster than those who did not. New work at the University of Buffalo assists athletes in maintaining their physical condition while recovering from head injury. Following a resting period of a minimum of three weeks, athletes begin a process of "regulated exercise," tailored to the individual. The authors of the study are optimistic about the results, and point out that their approach does not involve any medications, is cost-effective, and helps to reduce depression in patients. Underlying their approach is the hypothesis that regulated exercise helps to normalize cerebral blood flow, which may be dysfunctional in people with PCS.

Postconcussion Syndrome in Military Personnel

One common scenario that generates repeated head injury, from mild to moderate, is active military combat. From experiencing the effects of improvised explosive devices (IEDs), car bombs, automatic weapons fires, vehicle crashes, war is tough on the body and the brain. Military doctors estimate that 10% to 20% of soldiers returning from Iraq or Afghanistan suffer from PCS. At the higher end, that means more than 300,000 people with PCS–300,000 people needing ongoing medical care, perhaps for years, at a conservative estimate of $554 million dollars. In fact, PCS is so characteristic of modern warfare that the military is now giving soldiers a "brain test" before deployment, assessing basic abilities in math, identifying symbols, and measuring accuracy. These same tests will then be used to reassess returning soldiers who have suffered a concussion or other head injury in an effort to better diagnose, understand, and treat brain injuries. If a neurological deficit is identified, targeted therapy may help to retrain the soldier's brain to overcome cognitive problems.

SYMPTOMS

Symptoms range from minor to moderate headaches and dizziness to memory loss or even vision changes. It is hard sometimes for soldiers caught up in carrying out their stressful jobs to realize exactly how they've been affected. Sometimes it takes an observant partner to recognize the change and encourage the PCS patient to get help. One study involving more than 2,500 soldiers with mild PCS showed that these soldiers were more likely to suffer from poor health, missed work days, and postconcussive symptoms. Problems with balance, vision, and depression, along with posttraumatic stress disorder (PTSD) are common.

PTH appears to be a pervasive problem: One study found that nearly 70% of people who suffer from mild PCS report PTH. Recent studies done with soldiers returning from the Middle East found that migraine prevalence in this group was nearly twice that of the general population. They also find higher rates of PTSD, depression, and anxiety in returning soldiers. In response, The National Headache Foundation put together the War Veterans Health Resource Initiative to provide veterans with comprehensive information on managing headache and migraine, as well other aspects of health care in civilian life.

All of us in every walk of life have the potential to suffer a head injury that could lead to PTH or other serious health problems. The Brain Injury Resource Center maintains a website that offers a "Brain Injury Checklist" of more than 100 possible symptoms that can be scored to determine the likelihood of TBI and posttraumatic symptoms: www.headinjury.com/checktbi.htm

The next chapter looks at the important role inflammation plays in many chronic diseases, including some common autoimmune disorders, and how this can contribute to headache symptoms.

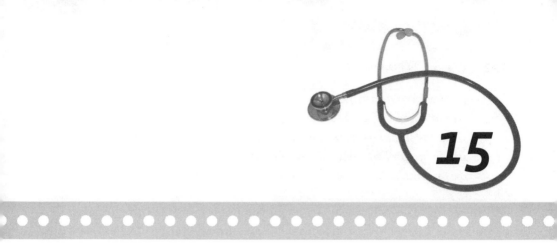

Inflammatory and Noninfectious Diseases and Headaches

Most people don't know that headaches can be caused by inflammation related to an autoimmune disorder. But if you have temporal arteritis, or an inflammation of the temporal artery, you know this only too well. What's more, the severe pain can radiate into other areas of the face and jaw. Visual disturbances are part of the picture, too, which I find to be really scary, and I'm really worried about losing my vision if I'm not very careful. Sometimes I feel dizzy and nauseous, too. But from the outside, most people don't have any idea what I am dealing with—it's an "invisible illness." I've had to go through a lot just to be diagnosed. First I was told it was from muscle spasms, then migraines. Finally I was correctly diagnosed, but then discovered that the treatment, using prednisone, caused other problems. I decided to be proactive and do everything I could for my overall health, including following an antiinflammatory diet. This seemed to make sense to me since the problem is "inflammation," and it has helped. Getting regular exercise and avoiding stress seem to also contribute to my ability to avoid these painful episodes. But it requires an ongoing commitment to stay healthy. MARIA

In recent years, we've learned about the important role inflammation plays in many chronic diseases. We also know that headaches are a common symptom in many inflammatory disorders. In this chapter, I'll present a brief overview of headaches in a range of chronic diseases.

Lupus

Lupus is a complex autoimmune disorder that affects an estimated 500,000 to 1,000,000 or more people in the United States. In autoimmune diseases, the body's immune system targets the body's own tissues, and in the case of lupus, multiple organs and systems throughout the body.

SYMPTOMS

Symptoms can include

- Fatigue
- Joint and muscles pain
- Low-grade fever
- Eye irritation
- Mild to moderate patchy hair loss
- Depression
- Headache

If lupus attacks the kidneys, fatal kidney damage can result. The cause or causes of lupus are unknown and may include genetic, environmental, and hormonal factors. Women are affected more often than men.

In addition to the abnormalities mentioned above, lupus affects blood vessels throughout the body. In about 20% of patients, inflammation of vessels in the brain is thought to cause "lupus headache," with symptoms typically resembling migraine: pulsating pain

What Nurses Know...

Autoimmune disorders tend to cluster, and there is a higher incidence of lupus among people with some other autoimmune disorders, including celiac disease, Sjogren's syndrome, and the inflammatory bladder disorder interstitial cystitis (IC/PBS).

lasting up to 4 hours, visual disturbances, nausea, and vomiting. Problems with the brain's functions governing thought and behavior are also present in up to half of lupus patients at some point in their illness, including confusion, memory impairment, and difficulty with speech and expressing thoughts. More alarming neurological symptoms such as seizures or signs of psychological disturbance may affect lupus patients. These symptoms may be due to a disturbance in blood flow in the brain. Lupus patients can also experience headaches from increased intracranial pressure.

Some neurologists feel that the headaches lupus patients experience are, in fact, primary headaches—either migraine or tension headaches, and they do not believe in the concept of a separate "lupus headache." A 2011 study published in *Headache* found that lupus patients may suffer higher levels of tension-type headache (TTH) but not migraine. And a recent meta-study published in *Brain* found no difference in the prevalence of TTH or migraine without aura between lupus patients and those in the general population. However, migraine with aura *is* thought to be more prevalent among lupus patients than in the general population. Given the overlap between migraine with aura and lupus, the possibility of undiagnosed lupus should be considered in migraine patients with prolonged or atypical symptoms, especially in those with family history or other risk factors for lupus.

TREATMENT

Lupus is treated with drugs to suppress the immune system and by closely monitoring patients for health crises. Mild lupus headaches may respond to over-the-counter (OTC) analgesics. Moderate or

What Nurses Know...

Lupus patients who have "Raynaud's phenomenon," with greatly restricted blood flow to the hands and fingers, and those patients who are positive for antiphosoholipid antibodies (APS)—sticky blood proteins that increase the risk of blood clots—may be at higher risk for lupus headache. Research has also shown that adult lupus patients who have suffered strokes often report having a history of migraine headaches as teens.

severe lupus headaches are treated with acute migraine medications including triptans, sometimes with the addition of corticosteroids to reduce lupus-related inflammation. Preventive medications may be used for patients who experience frequent migraine-like headaches, including antiseizure medications like Topamax, Depakote, and Neurontin, as well as antidepressants and drugs used to prevent high blood pressure.

Lupus patients require regular medical care, including access to medications, regular dental care, and eye exams. They also need guidance on exercise, diet, stress reduction, proper rest, and avoiding common migraine triggers. Following these guidelines can have powerful benefits for lupus patients.

Temporal Arteritis

Temporal arteritis, also known as giant-cell arteritis (GCA) is an autoimmune-driven inflammation of the blood vessels which affects nearly a quarter of a million people in the United States.

GCA can occur along with other autoimmune disorders, including lupus, rheumatoid arthritis, and polymyalgia rheumatic (a condition involving chronic pain in the shoulders and hips, and morning stiffness), and may be caused by the same underlying chronic inflammatory process. It usually affects the medium and large arteries of the head, causing pain in the temple area when it inflames the temporal artery. GCA is a form of vasculitis, or inflammation of the blood vessels, that affects more women than men. GCA usually affects people over fifty and more often seems to affect those of Scandinavian descent.

SYMPTOMS

GCA causes a range of symptoms including:

- Joint pain
- Fever
- Scalp tenderness
- Facial pain
- Pain in the jaw and tongue
- Blurry vision
- Ringing in the ears
- Headache

Visual symptoms are caused by inflammation of the ophthalmic artery, and can progress to loss of vision. This can happen abruptly and is considered a medical emergency. But headache with tenderness and a visible, slight swelling in the temple area is usually prominent both at diagnosis and at times of relapse. Even gentle touch of the head is uncomfortable and may aggravate symptoms.

DIAGNOSIS

GCA is uncommon the general population and its varied symptoms can make diagnosis difficult. But it may be of value to know that in patients over age 65, 16% of patients seeking medical care for a "fever of unknown origin" are ultimately diagnosed with GCA—a far higher percentage than in younger patients with similar symptoms. Levels of inflammatory markers may be raised. A complete blood count may reveal anemia and elevated platelets, but a normal white blood cell count. Examining the temporal artery with ultrasound may yield a "halo sign," which is indicative of inflammation surrounding the artery, but recent innovations such as high resolution MRI with contrast can diagnose temporal arteritis with a greater degree of specificity and sensitivity.

TREATMENT

Corticosteroids, usually high-dose prednisone (40-60 mg twice daily), is the treatment of choice and must be started quickly to reduce the risk of damage to the eye. Most patients begin to respond within a few days and recovery can be quite rapid. The dose of prednisone can be decreased after several weeks and tapered slowly over many months. Johns Hopkins Medical Center is one of the research institutions investigating the use of methotrexate, but its usefulness seems to still be debated. Low-dose aspirin appears to lower the risk of eye-related complications, especially in patients with an increased risk of blood clots, and some experts recommend that all patients with GCA take low-dose aspirin (81 mg "baby" aspirin).

With timely and appropriate treatment, GCA is a manageable disease, but relapses and recurrences are common. In a recent study involving 174 patients with confirmed GCA, roughly 41% of patients relapsed within 1 year, and the best predictor of relapse was the presence of iron-deficiency anemia at the time of diagnosis. For unknown reasons GCA tends to plague patients on and off for several years and then subside.

Chronic Fatigue Syndrome and Headaches

Tens of millions of people in the United States suffer from fatigue-related illnesses and more than 1 million have been officially diagnosed with chronic fatigue syndrome. Called CFS in some countries it is also known as Myalgic Encephalomyelitis (ME), or CFS/ME.

What Nurses Know...

Corticosteroids like prednisone can have significant side effects so be sure to discuss these with your doctor and pharmacist. Never stop taking these drugs abruptly and don't change the dose unless advised to do so by a health professional.

Women are affected four times as often as men, and the disease onset is typically after age 40, although it can occur much earlier in life—even in children. Many cases of CFS begin with a flu-like illness and symptoms continue to resemble those of a lingering virus, which may perhaps be why researchers and clinicians often look for a viral cause. But in many patients the search is not conclusive.

People living with CFS often complain of headaches, and patients may describe a new type of headache (similar to TTH), a new pattern, or increased severity of an existing headache.

TREATMENT

After excluding or treating other causes of fatigue, such as anemia or thyroid problems, treatment is focused on providing symptomatic relief and supporting patients in making healthy lifestyle changes. CFS-related headaches may respond to OTC analgesics or comfort treatments such as warm or cool packs. Drugs like Lyrica (pregabalin) may help if headaches become severe or chronic. The medications Fludrocortisone, a corticosteroid, and low-dose Naltrexone have both been used in treating CFS. Naltrexone blocks opioid receptors in the brain while stimulating the body to produce its own opioids—the endorphins. Experimental treatment with Naltrexone has been encouraging.

Nexavir (kutapressin) is another drug that has been trialed on CFS patients. It is an animal-derived product which may have strong antiviral and immune-modulating activity. Kutapressin has been

What Nurses Know...

CFS is a frustrating disorder for which we still have no known single cause or cure—although the search continues. For a period of time, this syndrome was linked to the retro-virus XMRV and some patients were treated with antiviral drugs, but a study released in 2011 showed that earlier studies were flawed and that the causal relationship between XMRV and CFS isn't clear.

tested against human herpesvirus-6 in in vitro studies, and against Epstein-Barr Virus (EBV) in patients with CFS. Kutapressin is usually given by injection.

Nutraceutical supplements that help boost mitochondrial energy production, such as Coenzyme Q-10 and D-Ribose, have been used in the treatment of CFS.

Some patients benefit from physical therapy, stretching or yoga practice, nutritional supplements, massage, an antiinflammatory or "Mediterranean" diet, and an exercise program geared toward moderate conditioning. Other positive lifestyle changes include reducing caffeine, alcohol, and nicotine use, reducing stress, engaging in CAM therapies, and getting adequate rest. In fact, many patients and their doctors feel that improving sleep is key to easing fatigue in both CFS and fibromyalgia (FM). Making the bedroom a restful, serene place used only for sleep and taking time to relax and unwind before bedtime may help.

Fibromyalgia and Headaches

A disorder that frequently coexists with CFS is FM, a chronic pain sensitization disorder affecting at least 5 million U.S. adults. Central sensitization disorders are thought to arise from abnormal changes in the nerve pathways in the brain and spinal cord, resulting in increased sensitivity to pain signals. FM is characterized by fatigue and nonrestful sleep, as in CFS, but this disorder also involves profound tenderness in the muscles and fascia of the body and a pattern of "hypersensitive" tender points in specific areas usually occurring symmetrically on both sides of the body. FM patients feel pain in response to light pressure, when most people would not.

What Nurses Know...

Sleep brightens a patient's outlook, helps patients cope better with pain, and improves concentration and energy level. Restful sleep is also necessary for the damaged immune system to recover.

FM patients also commonly suffer from three types of headaches: TTH, migraines, and, most often, combination tension/migraine headaches. Headaches may be influenced by a variety of factors: sleep disturbances, stress, muscle tension, and fatigue, as well as referred pain from trigger points in the neck, head, and shoulders. Headaches may also be due to side-effects from medications or from hormonal fluctuations in women.

More than half of FM patients say they suffer from frequent headaches including migraines, and research shows that there is a close association between FM and chronic headaches. The American Council for Headache Education (ACHE) reports that "Patients with FM share many features with chronic headache patients. Similar to migraine, FM occurs most commonly in women of childbearing age, with women affected seven times more often than men." One study found that 36% of chronic migraine patients had FM, while no more than 5% of the general population suffers from this disorder. Patients who had both chronic migraines and FM reported the most severe pain and depression. Another study found that 42% of chronic headache patients had the characteristic FM tender points. It seems likely that abnormalities in the regulation of the neurotransmitter serotonin and increased levels of substance P, an inflammatory neurotransmitter associated with pain, may contribute to nervous system overstimulation and hypersensitivity in both FM and migraine. Other studies have shown both FM patients and migraineurs have decreased levels of magnesium, which can be remedied by oral supplementation or other means.

TREATMENT

Medications used to treat FM include neuropathic pain modulators like Lyrica (pregabalin), and newer antidepressants such as Cymbalta (duloxetine) and the new FM management drug Savella (milnacipran), a selective serotonin and norepinephrine reuptake inhibitor (SNRI), which has not been approved to treat depression. Treating headaches in FM, as in standard treatment of migraine, includes medications such as triptans, ergot alkaloids, calcium channel blockers, and beta blockers, along with preventive medications, dietary modifications, and lifestyle changes. It has been reported that medications and therapies used to treat headache often also help relieve symptoms of FM.

Multiple Sclerosis and Headaches

Multiple sclerosis (MS) is a chronic autoimmune disorder that affects the nervous system, causing inflammation and damage to the protective myelin sheath surrounding the nerves of the brain and spinal cord. There is some disagreement as to whether headaches are a common symptom of MS, but many patients insist that they never had headaches prior to developing the disease and many patients report particular types of headache symptoms associated with MS.

Damage to the nerves involved creates a range of common symptoms, including fatigue, vision problems, impaired coordination, dizziness, pain, muscle spasticity, headaches, and depression.

According to studies, roughly 58% of MS patients experience chronic or recurring migraine-like headaches and a third of MS patients have a prior diagnosis of migraine. Both of these statistics are much higher than would be expected in the general population. MS patients are more prone to at least three other types of headaches: cluster-like headaches, tension headaches, and ocular migraines and/or optic neuritis. Headaches in MS can be also caused by the same factors that trigger headaches in the general population, such as increased stress, tension, dehydration, and environmental factors. Headaches specific to MS patients have

What Nurses Know...

What causes the body's immune system to attack the myelin sheath remains unknown. But stress, as well as some dietary factors, including gluten grains, dairy, eggs, and yeast, seems to trigger attacks of symptoms. Like other autoimmune disorders, there are usually flares and remissions of symptoms in MS.

many possible causes, including lesions in areas of the brain where the headache originates, disease-related depression, and reactions to some MS medications. Forms of interferon (Rebif), and medications such as Betaseron and Avonex can increase the frequency and severity of headaches in MS patients. Likewise, medications used to treat fatigue in MS, including Provigil and Symmetrel, list headaches as a side effect.

Migraine in MS is often preceded by visual aura and fatigue. It is a typical throbbing headache accompanied by sensitivity to light and sound, nausea, and vomiting, lasting from about 4 to 12 hours. Patients may experience some continued discomfort during the postdromal period following the headache. Some may experience prolonged fatigue and dizziness that may temporarily worsen mobility problems and make managing their disease more difficult. Migraine headaches are more common in people with the relapsing-remitting form of the disease, which affects 85% of people with MS.

There is also an association between cluster headache in MS and lesions in the area of the brain where the trigeminal nerve (5th cranial nerve) originates. Cluster headaches tend to follow the same pattern as they do in those without MS, reaching a peak within a very short time. Pain and visual symptoms are confined to one side of the face or behind one eye, and reoccur regularly at about the same time each day—at bedtime or shortly after falling asleep. They may be very brief, lasting only about 15 minutes, or in some patients, lasting up to 3 hours, with less residual discomfort than with migraine. Headache cluster periods can result in increased anxiety and sleep difficulties in MS patients.

Tension-type headaches can also occur in MS patients, often building up gradually in late afternoon, creating a band of pressure surrounding the head. There is often associated upper neck and shoulder tension, and while not excruciating, these headaches result in constant, nagging pain lasting from less than an hour to a full day. However, tension-type headaches usually respond well to OTC analgesics, relaxation, and restful sleep.

The recent large-scale Nurses' Health Study II showed that women with a diagnosis of migraine were 47% more likely to develop MS than women without migraine, regardless of age, vitamin D level, body mass index, history of smoking, and geographical location. This study gave us an important look into the association between MS and migraine, but the author, Dr. Ilya Kister, of the New York University School of Medicine, has stressed that more research is needed to know if migraine is a risk factor for MS, or if it is a symptom of MS. Writer and MS patient Ann Pietrangelo has remarked, "Migraines and MS share common ground. They are both widely misunderstood and often dismissed as psychological in nature. They are both more common to women than men. They both will change the way you live your life."

TREATMENT

MS treatments include interferon-based medications, Rebif, Betaseron, and Avonex. Fatigue in MS may be treated with Provigil and Symmetrel. Headaches in MS are treated with standard headache medications. Massage therapy may be a useful adjunct to MS care, especially for patients who suffer frequent tension headaches.

Optic Neuritis—Headache and Visual Symptoms in MS

A serious eye-related condition, which also causes headaches, affects a significant number of MS patients: Optic Neuritis (ON). When a nerve becomes inflamed the condition is called "neuritis". ON is an inflammation of the optic nerve, cranial nerve 2, which relays light and visual image messages between the retina of the eye and the brain. These messages are then translated in the visual cortex to become what we recognize as vision. ON is associated with MS, Lupus, and other autoimmune disorders, and with serious infections like meningitis. Other conditions that can cause decreased blood flow to the optic nerve, including cranial arteritis (an inflammation of the lining of cranial arteries) and diabetes (a metabolic disorder involving problems with blood sugar regulation), can lead to ON. This disorder affects more women than men, with a mean age of onset of 30 to 35. Total prevalence is 115 cases per 100,000 persons.

SYMPTOMS

ON can rapidly reduce normal vision in the affected eye, causing eye pain, visual distortions, changes in the pupil's reaction to light, and loss of color vision. This disorder is associated with one-sided headaches that worsen with eye movements such as looking up, down, or to the side. Symptoms may also be worsened by heat or exercise.

In an early study on ON, 16% of patients described their symptoms as a headache centering on the affected eye and in another 14% it was described as a generalized dull headache. A large majority of patients also report vision loss and eye pain.

DIAGNOSIS

Your doctor or eye doctor can diagnose ON by evaluating your symptoms, looking into your eye with an ophthalmoscope for visible swelling of the optic nerve and enlargement of the surrounding blood vessels—or by viewing the results of MRI views of the brain that show the optic nerve. A thorough workup, including MRI with special contrast, is essential in a first episode of ON in order to look for abnormalities in the brain that can cause visual symptoms.

TREATMENT

When an acute infectious cause for the disease can be found and treated, patients have a good chance of recovery. When the condition is associated with a chronic condition such as an autoimmune disease like MS or lupus, patients' chances of total recovery are not as good.

Studies examining past medical history of MS patients have shown that roughly half of those ages 15 to 50 who experience ON will eventually go on to develop MS within 15 years, and 15% to 20% of MS patients report ON as their initial MS symptom. Thus, ON has become one of the conditions linked to the onset of MS. When MS is diagnosed as a result of ON as an initial symptom, treatment with immune-suppressive medications or other treatments may decrease the risk of future attacks of both MS and ON.

Depending on the cause, ON can sometimes clear on its own within a few weeks, or it may be cautiously treated with IV corticosteroids. ON may reoccur in conjunction with disease flares. Complications can include permanent vision loss and side-effects from corticoster-oids. Contact your doctor if you experience any of the following:

- New symptoms of eye pain or changes in vision.
- Worsening symptoms of pre-existing ON: new eye pain, worsening vision, or symptoms that don't improve with your usual treatment.
- Unusual neurological and motor symptoms including numbness, weakness, or difficulty with coordination.

The next chapter discusses secondary headaches caused by infec-tious diseases, including some that cause devastating changes to the protective immune system.

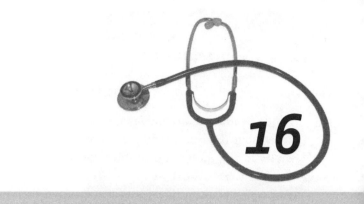

Headaches
and Infectious Diseases

I've had sinus headaches all my life, and every winter, at least one very long-lasting sinus infection requiring treatment with antibiotics. My sinus headaches begin with a dull throbbing in the center of my forehead. There is a strong feeling of pressure, which is intensified if I bend over. My head feels heavy and my thinking is foggy. Everything seems like such an effort. Sometimes the pain seems to radiate into the sides of my nose or even behind my eyes. This winter, though, I have not had my usual sinus congestion that seems to lead to chronic sinus headaches and infections. I recently had testing done that showed an allergy to dairy products, and I have worked very hard to try to eliminate all sources of dairy from my diet. This seems to have cleared up my congestion, and also some digestive issues I was having. I still get nervous when I see those dark winter clouds begin to descend, but so far they have not brought with them my usual winter sinus headaches. CAROLYN

Sinus Headache

Sinus headaches are one example of secondary headaches caused by infectious disease. Many people complain of "sinus headaches," especially in the damp and cool winter months, and they are commonly treated with over-the-counter (OTC) analgesics and decongestants. But not all "sinus headaches" respond to these simple treatments, with good reason—they may actually be migraines, and I'll explain how to tell the difference.

WHO GETS THEM AND WHY?

In adults, there are four, symmetrically paired sinuses, which are small air-filled chambers located just behind the forehead, cheekbones, and bridge of the nose. They are lined with membranes that produce a thick mucous that drains out of the nose, helping to trap and expel harmful substances we've inhaled. Sinuses can become inflamed as a result of exposure to an ingested allergen like dairy protein, irritation from environmental allergens such as pollen and mold, or chemical irritation by breathing fumes or cigarette smoke. Sinuses can also become inflamed and congested as a result of infection—a condition known as "rhinosinusitis"—which may affect as many as 37 million Americans. When any of these situations occurs, we may develop a headache, along with other symptoms such as a runny or congested nose, or a feeling of fullness in or "plugging up" of the ears. People with asthma, nasal polyps, dust-, mold-, pollen-allergies, or weakened immune systems may be especially prone to rhinosinusitis. But one of the most frequent causes of rhinosinusitis is the common cold, or upper respiratory virus. If you don't feel better after a week or so following a head cold, see your doctor—especially if you develop symptoms of a persistent sinus headache that cannot be relieved by using OTC headache medications, rest, and comfort measures such as warm compresses applied over the sinuses.

SYMPTOMS

Sinus headache pain tends to be deep and constant, and to worsen when lying down or bending over. Pressing on the face over the sinuses may cause discomfort, and facial puffiness may be visible under the eyes and on either side of the nose. Pain and/or pressure may be felt around the eye sockets, brow region, forehead, cheeks, and even the upper jaws and teeth. If the headache is related to rhinosinusitis there may be thick, yellow-green or blood-tinged mucous drainage from the nose, throat irritation, and a decreased sense of smell. A fever is often present, and patients may feel profound fatigue and malaise. True sinus headaches tend to be worse upon awakening, and to clear up as the day progresses and the sinuses have the assistance of gravity to drain.

DIAGNOSIS

Your doctor may ask you questions that help to distinguish true sinus headaches from migraines, as the two disorders are very easy to confuse. In fact, a large study showed that the majority of suspected sinus headaches met the ICHD-II criteria for migraine and responded well to triptans—typical migraine medications. These two headaches share many features such as pain that worsens when bending forward, a throbbing quality, and nasal congestion. Similarly, studies have also shown that migraines are more common in people with allergic rhinitis, which is often interpreted as a "sinus problem." But *key* differences are that sinus headaches rarely are accompanied by nausea or vomiting and are not associated with sensitivity to light or sound. Your doctor may also inquire about your recent health history and whether you've had a recent cold or hay fever. Further diagnosis of sinus headache involves a physical examination, with special attention to the nasal passages and mucous membranes. Your doctor may use a special instrument to look up your nose and may swab your nose with a large cotton-tipped applicator to culture your nasal drainage for microorganisms. Imaging, including facial x-ray, CT, or MRI may be done to determine if your sinuses are blocked. Sinus blockages can sometimes result in an abscess, which can lead to dangerous complications. If you suffer from chronic sinusitis, your doctor may order allergy tests or refer you to a doctor who specializes in ear, nose, and throat disorders—an ENT, or otolaryngologist.

TREATMENT

Goals of treatment are to treat the bacterial infection, reduce swelling in the nasal passages, and drain the sinuses. Rhinosinusitis is treated with oral antibiotics.

If OTC decongestants are not enough to relieve inflammation your doctor may prescribe a corticosteroid or saline nasal spray. Take care not to overuse such medications, as some can be habit-forming and can lead to complications including chronic daily headache. Pain may be managed using OTC analgesics like acetaminophen or nonsteroidal antiinflammatory drugs (NSAIDs). In some cases, there are structural abnormalities that make it difficult for the sinuses to drain properly, so corrective surgery is sometimes needed. If pain continues after a proper course of treatment with antibiotics and any other sinus symptoms subside, your doctor may reconsider your diagnosis: Migraine or tension-type headache are strong possibilities.

Pregnant women may want to try herbal or nondrug treatments such as capsaicin-based nasal sprays, steam inhalation with eucalyptus, peppermint, or thyme, or aromatherapy with the traditional Chinese medicine remedies magnolia and "white flower oil."

PREVENTION

Good hand-washing is helpful and is especially important if you are a health care professional or work with young children. Using an indoor

What Nurses Know...

Antibiotics can be given orally, in nebulizer form—aerosolized and breathed in through the nose—or intravenously. Remember, you must finish all of the prescribed antibiotics in order to kill off all of the microorganisms causing the infection. If you do not finish your prescribed medicine the infection can come back, perhaps with more serious symptoms.

room air humidifier can help moisten and soothe irritated nasal passages, while using a high efficiency particulate air (HEPA) filter can help remove potential irritants from the air. Avoiding tobacco smoke, even second-hand smoke, is a very good idea.

Herbal treatments include the antiinflammatory enzyme bromelain and the bioflavinoid quercetin. "Sinupret," a compound herbal formula made up of the immune stimulant *Sambucus nigra* (Elderberry) and five other herbs, was found to be more effective than placebo in relieving sinus symptoms. A tea made from white willow bark (*Salix* sp.) is also helpful in alleviating headache pain. Acupuncture, using specific points to open the sinuses, for nasal congestion, or for blocked ears—as well as chiropractic and homeopathy treatments—has also been used to treat sinus headaches. Finally, simple facial self-massage may be comforting and help to boost circulation.

What Nurses Know...

Many people prone to sinus problems find regular irrigation of the nasal passages with a mild, warm, saline solution can be a helpful preventive strategy. You can make up a simple saline solution by mixing tsp. sea salt in one-cup warm water and use an old-fashioned bulb syringe or a "netti-pot"—a small pot with a narrow spout that fits the nostrils. A method that is very simple and safe to use is to pour the salt solution into your clean, cupped hand, tilt your head at an angle down to your raised hand, and inhale through one nostril while pinching the other nostril off with a finger. Tucking the chin downward helps to close off the airway and helps prevent the risk of choking. Using any of these methods, the solution should run through your nasal passages and run out into your mouth where you can spit it out. Use nonchlorinated spring water or distilled water. If you have an ear infection, you should not irrigate the sinuses until the ear infection is gone.

The Epstein-Barr Virus and New Daily Persistent Headache

The Epstein-Barr virus (EBV) causes a flu-like illness called infectious mononucleosis, or "mono," which quite often can later lead to serious complications. This common virus related to the herpes viruses is known to affect a large number of people each year, although most of them recover without lingering symptoms. But in some patients, EBV can persist in the body, where it can activate the immune system, causing central nervous system damage. It is thought that EBV can become "reactivated" by stress or some other unknown factor, which may lead to these associated disorders later in life.

In the past few years, this common virus has also been linked to the development of new daily persistent headache (NDPH), a sub-type of chronic daily headache.

NDPH is defined as a daily unremitting headache occurring in people without a prior history of headache. More than twice as many women than men are diagnosed with NDPH, and women tend to be diagnosed earlier. Symptoms may resemble either migraine or tension-type headache, but pain is usually felt in both sides of the head, and nausea and vomiting occur less frequently than in migraine.

A diagnosis of NDPH is made after first ruling out other possible causes for daily headache:

- Headaches caused by trauma
- Active viral infection
- Spinal headache from the leakage of cerebrospinal fluid
- Medication overuse headache

Official diagnostic criteria state that NDPH patients must have daily pain lasting longer than 4 hours each day, and the daily or near-daily headache must have been present for at least 2 months.

The link between NDPH and past infection with EBV is strong. One study with 32 NDPH patients found that 84% had positive titers for active EBV infection, versus only 25% of controls. Certainly any patient with NDPH needs to have a thorough neurological workup, which may include an MRI with contrast, complete blood work, and titers to rule out both EBV and Lyme disease, which can cause similar symptoms, including unrelenting fatigue.

What Nurses Know...

Lyme disease is an infection caused by a type of bacteria carried by ticks, and it can lead to symptoms anywhere in the body. Lyme disease can cause symptoms including weakness, fatigue, sensitivity to light, visual symptoms, and severe, persistent, new onset headaches, somewhat resembling migraine. But in Lyme disease, the headache may be a frontal headache affecting both sides of the head. Lyme patients are sometimes referred to a chronic pain specialist or physician specializing in the treatment of infectious diseases.

TREATMENT

If no definitive cause for NDPH can be found, then symptomatic treatment proceeds as for chronic daily headache, with antiinflammatories, antidepressants, and other medications. Some NDPHs eventually subside, while others persist, and may even be resistant to treatment.

People who wish to investigate alternative treatment for EBV might look into herbal treatments with the guidance of a specialist in botanical medicine. One treatment widely discussed is olive leaf extract, which may have antiviral properties. Side effects of use can include symptoms of detoxification, such as fatigue, diarrhea,

What Nurses Know...

Some cases of NDPH have resolved when patients were successfully treated for an underactive thyroid. Overall, patients with NDPH have reason to be somewhat optimistic because long-term studies have shown that after two years 86% of men and 73% of women saw an end to their NDPH.

headaches, or flu-like symptoms, but these are temporary. The safety of olive leaf extract in pregnant or nursing women isn't known.

Herpes-Virus Varicella Zoster—Shingles and Chronic Headache

You may have contracted the viral illness chickenpox as a child—9 out of 10 U.S. adults have. The varicella zoster virus (VZV) that causes this childhood illness (which also affects some adults) remains dormant in the body throughout life, but it can become active again, causing the painful, blistering rash known as shingles. This painful condition, affecting up to 1,000,000 people a year in the United States, frequently makes its appearance on one side of the abdomen, or down one arm or one leg. Less frequently it can appear on the head or face, and can affect the eye. Those with shingles-associated eye pain should seek *immediate medical treatment*—shingles of the eye can cause scarring that leads to blindness and can increase the risk of developing glaucoma. Shingles also causes headaches, as well as a complication known as *postherpetic neuralgia* (PHN), which may lead to chronic pain.

SYMPTOMS

The shingles virus travels along a nerve pathway. Patients can experience odd neurological symptoms such as localized pain, itching, tingling, or numbness, along with tiny fluid-filled blisters known as vesicles. Patients may also have flu-like symptoms without fever, which may precede the appearance of blisters clustered in a rash-like pattern. Patients should avoid scratching blisters open, which can increase the risk for secondary infection and scarring. Sensitivity to light (photophobia) may be present, and shingles can produce *severe migraine-like headaches*, especially when the outbreak is on the head or face.

DIAGNOSIS

Diagnosing shingles isn't usually difficult: Shingles is fairly common, most doctors have seen it many times in many forms, and no special tests are necessary. Diagnosis is based on a thorough patient exam and ruling out other possible conditions. You may be asked if you have ever had chicken pox. If you suspect shingles, call your doctor's office. Your doctor can perform a blood test to check for antibodies to VZV to determine whether you've had chickenpox; sometimes the childhood illness is very mild or there isn't a family medical history. If you suspect shingles, avoid contact with the general public, including your doctor's office waiting room. During the period when the fluid-filled blisters are present, *shingles is considered to be contagious*! Pregnant women, adults who have never had chicken pox, and persons with weak immune systems need to be especially careful to avoid exposure. As a health care professional, if you have never had chicken pox, you should request a change in assignment; if you are or could be pregnant, you need to *insist* on it. Health professionals who work with seniors are at increased risk, as shingles most often affects those over age 60.

TREATMENT

Beyond offering supportive care, in many cases it may be necessary to treat pain or itching. Physicians may also prescribe an antiviral drug such as acyclovir or famciclovir, especially in immune-compromised patients, to help to shorten the course of active shingles eruptions and prevent life-threatening complications.

SHINGLES COMPLICATIONS

Older patients and those with diabetes, cancer, HIV/AIDS, or a history of organ transplant are at increased risk for developing complications. The most common complication is PHN, the mild to severe long-term pain that follows a shingles outbreak in about 10% to 15% of patients. PHN causes burning, searing pain along the affected nerve pathway long after the rash has healed and other symptoms have subsided. Nerve pain may wax and wane unpredictably, and may worsen at night. If the affected nerve is on the head or face, *persistent headache*, facial pain, or cutaneous allodynia (which can also be present in other headache disorders) may occur. The affected skin is hypersensitive, even to the movement of air across the skin, hair brushing, and the touch of clothing. Damaged nerves may also cause temporary muscle weakness.

Your doctor can diagnose PHN if such symptoms of chronic pain develop *after* a shingles outbreak. Your doctor may refer you to a neurologist who specializes in the treatment of chronic pain. A combination of treatments may include oral medications such as tricyclic antidepressants, antiseizure medications such as Neurontin (gabapentin) or Lyrica (pregabalin), or a controlled course of narcotics. Topical lidocaine patches may be cut and applied to fit the affected area. Some patients have had good results with capsaicin cream (Capzasin-P, Zostrix), applied with gloves, but it should never be used near the eyes or on broken or irritated skin. Topical aspirin creams may also help reduce skin sensitivity.

A new vaccine for shingles prevention has been approved for use in those over age 60: Zostavax reduces the risk of developing both shingles and PHN, although it is not useful in the treatment of *active* shingles. Half of persons aged 80 or older will experience at least one attack of shingles—and these patients tend to have a higher risk for long-term complications such as PHN, so the shingles vaccine is worth considering in your later years. However, people with weakened immune systems cannot take the vaccine, which is made from the live virus.

Viral meningitis is another complication that (rarely) may follow a shingles outbreak. Although this disorder affects less than 1% of patients with shingles, it can be devastatingly painful, with extremely severe constant headache, sensitivity to light, muscle aches, and fever. Meningitis related to shingles is *viral*, not bacterial, so antibiotics are not effective and the illness must run its course—usually resulting in recovery within 7 to 10 days. Other viruses that can cause meningitis include herpes simplex, enterovirus, and the virus that causes the childhood illness "mumps." Meningitis patients can be made comfortable in a quiet, darkened room, and given pain medications and adequate hydration—especially important if fever is present.

HIV/AIDS and Headaches

HIV/AIDS is a viral, blood-borne, immunodeficiency disease caused by the HIV virus. At first thought to be a death sentence in those people who have been diagnosed, HIV/AIDS is now manageable, albeit with intensive and expensive medical intervention. More than 1 million people in the United States are currently living with HIV/AIDS. Both men and women are affected, and children can contract the virus through transmission in utero. Clearly, *prevention* is the key to reducing the impact of HIV/AIDS around the globe.

HIV weakens the immune system by destroying a specific type of white blood cell (CD4) that helps the body fight disease. HIV can exist in your body for many years before progressing to AIDS, the advanced form of the disease.

SYMPTOMS

You may already be familiar with some of the symptoms of HIV/AIDS, such as weight loss, fatigue, and susceptibility to opportunistic infections, but headaches are also common. They can be primary headaches such as migraine or tension headaches that can occur in anyone, or secondary headaches due to HIV/AIDS-related conditions. It is very common to experience a headache, along with fatigue, during the initial acute flu-like syndrome that affects up to 93% of individuals, beginning roughly 2 to 4 weeks following exposure to the virus. Headaches in HIV/AIDS can be a result of fever related to the systemic viral infection, or headaches can be present along with more serious symptoms of acute lymphocytic meningitis, including pain behind the eyes, extreme sensitivity to light and sound, and stiff neck. Other secondary HIV/AIDS-related headaches can occur as a result of the opportunistic infections and cancers to which patients are most susceptible: cryptococcal meningitis, toxoplasma encephalitis, and primary lymphoma of the central nervous system. Headaches resulting from meningitis tend to come on gradually, and are associated with fever, nausea, vomiting, and sensitivity to light; headaches resulting from masses or lesions have more variability in onset and symptoms, and are associated with neurological symptoms and confusion.

DIAGNOSIS

Diagnosis and treatment of headaches in HIV/AIDS patients are not easy. All patients presenting with new headaches need to have a thorough diagnostic workup, but patients with HIV/AIDS present special challenges. Failure to recognize very serious pathologies can lead to *life-threatening consequences*—even overlooking a sinus infection can lead to complications in an HIV/AIDS patient. A careful medical history and physical may be followed by an MRI to exclude infections and tumors in the brain. After ruling out serious problems, HIV/AIDS patients with persistent headaches are commonly diagnosed with a form of migraine headache to which they may be especially at risk: immune-driven inflammation develops around the blood vessels in the brain, causing severe headaches.

Migraine is most prevalent, occurring in 76% of HIV/AIDS patients presenting with primary headaches. Tension-type headaches and cluster headaches affect 14% and 10%, respectively. Unfortunately, about *half of those suffering from migraines develop chronic daily headaches.* The use of multiple medications, depression, anxiety, and sleep disorders are also commonly associated with primary headaches in HIV/AIDS patients. As in other people with migraines, headaches can be triggered by environmental conditions, hormonal imbalances, specific trigger foods, and stress. Patients may also be sensitive to odors, light, noise, and drops in blood sugar.

In very ill HIV/AIDS patients, a lumbar puncture is often necessary to obtain a sample of cerebrospinal fluid in order to rule out a treatable infectious cause. A spinal headache may occasionally follow lumbar puncture, but these headaches usually are self-limiting or easily resolved with a tiny injected "patch" of the patient's own blood.

TREATMENT

Highly active antiretroviral treatment (HAART) is the standard of care for HIV/AIDS patients. Treatment for neuropathic pain, caused by damage or illness that affects the nervous system, is also an important consideration. Treatment may include a short course of oral steroid (prednisone), while chronic headaches may be treated with low-dose amitriptyline or another, less-sedating, antidepressant. With a physician's guidance, NSAIDs and plain aspirin may be safe to use as well. HIV/AIDS patients with recurrent or chronic headaches can also be treated with the same acute and preventive medications used in typical migraine treatment, but it is especially important for patients to work with the physician familiar with treating their underlying condition, rather than with an unfamiliar specialist: There are potential drug interactions between HIV/AIDS drugs and medications used to treat headaches, and some drugs used to treat HIV/AIDS, especially zidovudine, amprenavir, lopinavir/ritonavir, and efavirenz, are known to cause or increase the severity of headaches. Headache side effects may recede with continued medication use. If patients continue to suffer from zidovudine-induced headaches, it may be possible to switch to a different antiretroviral drug.

A 2003 study described a rare but dangerous drug interaction between ergotamine-derived drugs and protease-inhibitors—acute vasospasm and central nervous system problems including seizure. It is now recommended that HIV/AIDS patients taking protease inhibitors *avoid using ergot alkaloid medications* to treat migraine; certainly there are safer and readily available alternatives. The drug ritonavir can increase blood concentrations of headache medications, including analgesics, antidepressants, calcium channel blockers, and ergotamine. One common potential interaction is between zidovudine and Tylenol (acetaminophen—also an ingredient in combination headache medications), leading to decreased blood levels of zidovudine.

PREVENTION

Patients looking for natural alternatives in headache treatment might consider taking Vitamin B2 (riboflavin) as recommended by their physician for headache prevention. Avoiding tobacco use, limiting caffeine consumption, getting adequate restful sleep, and avoiding stress are important. Some HIV/AIDS patients may benefit from CAM therapies such as biofeedback or acupuncture.

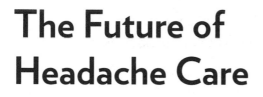

The Future of
Headache Care

*Until the triptans came on the market, I had a very hard
time managing my headaches. After trial and error, I finally
found a triptan that worked for me, but not 100% of the time.
It seems that I'm one of those people who have two different
types of migraines. My typical headache comes on slowly, and
if I take my medication early on in the headache, it's pretty
effective. But I have other headaches that arrive with what I
call a "ping" above my left eye, and these are much harder to
deal with. These headaches usually only responded to a shot
of Imitrex. So I was really excited about the new nasal spray
form of sumatriptan. Luckily, it worked well for me, and it
makes sense to have something that you can still use if you're
nauseous or vomiting. I can't wait to try the new patch they're
working on. "Big pharma" gets a lot of criticism, but I'm thankful that headache research is proceeding, because there are so
many people—millions of us—who can benefit.* MEG

Early treatments for severe headaches included simple analgesics like aspirin, still used today, and later ergotamine-based drugs. Beyond simple comfort measures, or opioid narcotics, there was little else to offer beyond drugs developed for other disorders—such as beta-blockers—until the past few decades. Then scientists focusing on the role of serotonin and 5-hydroxytryptamine receptor agonists developed a new class of highly effective drugs called triptans—the first medications to have a specific mechanism of action on migraine headaches and related disorders.

Possible New Treatments for Migraine and Other Headaches

First coming into use in the 1990s, triptans are now used in countries around the world, with total global sales of $3 billion dollars annually. Triptans truly revolutionized headache care, proving to be very useful in the treatment of:

- Migraine
- Cluster headache
- Some forms of tension-type headache

The best part is they don't have addictive qualities or potential for recreational abuse. In fact, some experts feel that the use of triptans has not yet reached its potential for treating large numbers of patients, and that many physicians still opt not to use triptans as a first-line treatment option for headache patients. For example, only 10% of migraine patients in one county in Denmark were treated with triptans. Research into new drug "delivery systems," which we'll discuss in more detail below, may enable more patients to benefit from triptans.

The Need for New Drug Approaches in Headache Prevention and Treatment

Few new classes of symptomatic migraine medications have been developed since the advent of triptans, and there are some groups of people who cannot tolerate the side-effects, or for whom triptans pose a heightened cardiovascular risk. Although triptans are effective in reducing the headache of migraine, they do not seem to be able to reduce allodynia, the skin hypersensitivity that accompanies this condition.

Another important need is for medications that can be used to treat chronic daily headache. Narcotic analgesics, medications containing caffeine, medications containing butalbital (Fioricet, Fiorinal), and several other medications have proven to be ineffective in treating very frequent headaches and have also been associated with the development of medication overuse (rebound) headache (MOH). Whether or not triptans also contribute to MOH seems to be conflicting, and I believe more research is needed. Some experts have pointed out that triptans work best when taken early in the headache, so continuing to take them repeatedly if a headache persists is ineffective—and there are better options, such as antiinflammatories. Overall, there remains a great need for additional approaches to treating problem headaches.

Targets of Current Research

A recent Danish study reviewed new targets for treatment in migraine attacks as a source for potential pharmaceutical development. Researchers are continuing to look closely at different mechanisms in the pathogenesis of migraine, including nitric oxide involvement, the action of calcitonin gene-related peptide (CGRP) receptors, the role of histamine in neurogenic inflammation, and the phenomenon of cortical spreading depression (CSD) in migraine. These different areas of research have been proven theoretically and have been investigated using human models.

NITRIC OXIDE IN MIGRAINE HEADACHE

The role of nitric oxide (NO) in migraine headache was the subject of several studies conducted in the 1990s. Researchers explored subjects' reactions to a form of nitroglycerin that easily penetrated the blood-brain barrier (GTN). They used this substance to deliver NO to areas both inside and outside the brain in both migraineurs and people without headaches. The researchers found that in people with migraines,

IV infusion of GTN caused a more immediate, intense headache. But what may be most interesting is that infusion of GTN also led to a delayed headache peaking 6 to 7 hours later—one that very closely resembled a typical attack of migraine without aura. This result was observed by researchers and also reported by patients. Most nonheadache patients, in contrast, experienced only the immediate headache, not the intense delayed headache that the migraineurs developed.

It has also been found that a compound that inhibited NO synthase, L-NMMA, effectively treated spontaneous migraine, confirming that NO plays a role throughout the duration of episodic migraine. This research has led to the development of another highly selective NOS inhibitor, GW274150, which has entered Phase II clinical trials. A related compound has entered Phase I trials. If these potential treatments proceed in development, new drugs with antiinflammatory action in migraine may become available for those who have been searching for answers.

CGRP IN MIGRAINE HEADACHE

We've known since the 1980s that CGRP helps to relax and dilate both the cranial and cerebral arteries. One thing that all migraine-provoking substances have in common is their ability to cause vasodilation. CGRP and its receptors have been found throughout nerve pathways in the brain and the dura mater. Further studies found increased CGRP in the external jugular vessels during acute migraine attacks. Also, intravenous infusion of CGRP triggered acute migraine or migraine-like symptoms in 8 out of 10 persons studied. Both of these findings have led to interest in searching for and developing a CGRP-agonist as a potential migraine treatment.

Now under development is a potential new group of medications that work by preventing CGRP from triggering blood vessel dilation. A compound known as BIBN4096BS, later called "olcegepant," was found to achieve a good response in treatment of acute migraine in Phase II clinical trials in a dose of about 5 mg, but olcegepant can only be administered by slow intravenous injection. Other companies are continuing to work on developing an orally administered CGRP receptor antagonist, and at least one compound, MK-0974, has now entered Phase III clinical trials, under the trade name "telcagepant."

HISTAMINE IN MIGRAINE HEADACHE

Studies done with another headache-provoking substance, histamine, have so far shown that blocking its action is not reliably effective in reducing or preventing migraine. Histamine causes more headaches in migraineurs than in those who don't get migraines, and histamine can lead to a delayed headache identical to spontaneous migraine. We also know that in experimental studies, blocking H-1 receptors with mepyramine, an antihistamine targeting the H1 receptor, was able to prevent specifically histamine-induced migraine headaches completely, in comparison to placebo. But unfortunately, H1 and H2 blockers have not proven to be effective in preventing spontaneous migraines in large numbers of people. Anecdotally, though, some patients have reported successful resolution of migraine following an intravenous cocktail including the antihistamine Benadryl (diphenhydramine), sometimes combined with other medications.

CSD IN MIGRAINE HEADACHE

CSD is a wave-like phenomenon of nerve cell depolarization that moves from its generation in the occipital cortex toward the front of the brain. Along with this "wave" comes a corresponding wave of hypoperfusion, or decreased blood flow, which has been observed during imaging of the brain in patients experiencing migraine with aura and may also be associated with migraine without aura. Currently, there are several pharmaceutical companies investigating this new theory along with potential drug treatments.

One promising new drug now called "tonabersat" is thought to work by helping to block CSD. This compound was first thought to be adaptable to symptomatic treatment of acute migraine, but so far studies have not yielded satisfactory results. However, tonabersat has shown some promise in migraine prevention, performing better than placebo. A new class of Serotonin 5-HT1F agonists, which do not have the vasoconstricting action of triptans, are entering Phase II studies. Additional targets of investigation include AMPA/kainate, TRPV1, and prostanoid EP4—any of which may lead to new potential drug treatments for migraine and other problem headaches. With new targets and the potential for therapeutic advances, the next era of antimigraine medications is on the horizon.

CSD is an important foundation of migraine headache theory and further study may offer another opportunity for intervention in patients with intractable migraine.

Transcranial Magnetic Stimulation (TMS) and Transcranial Direct Current Stimulation (tDCS) are two new therapies currently being tested in clinical trials for people suffering from migraine. These "pain-modulating devices," which work to interrupt signals in pain processing, have been applied in the treatment of other pain conditions. TMS uses weak electrical currents to induce a magnetic field, which then generates small currents of electricity in a specified area. In animal models, these electrical currents effectively block the wave of CSD that causes excitation of the neurons by more than 50%.

Many researchers now believe that spontaneous migraine attacks are generated in the brainstem, and it is thought that deep, neuro-modulatory brainstem structures may be a target site for TMS. One double-blind study of TMS for the treatment of acute migraine with aura showed very good results, with pain-free responses 2 hours after treatment, continuing to last for up to 48 hours. Similarly to the response of TMS, based on the results of low-intensity tDCS applied to the cerebral cortex, this new neuro-modulatory device is now in Phase II trials in patients with migraine with and without aura. If proven safe, TCS and tDCS offer alternatives for patients who cannot use vasoconstrictive medications such as ergotamines and triptans. A similar therapy called Occipital Nerve Stimulation was effective in a small number of patients with drug-resistant cluster headache, and six out of the eight patients receiving the new therapy said they would recommend it. New types of surgical treatments for cluster headache are also being refined.

New Headache Medications and New Ways to Take Them

Nausea and vomiting make it necessary to find alternate routes of providing medications so research is looking into new ways to deliver medicine. Current studies are underway on orally-inhaled dihydroergotamine (DHE) and transdermal skin patches of Imitrex (sumatriptan).

A new form of dihydroergotamine appears to be headed for FDA approval and may soon reach the market. Levadex, available in the form of an orally inhaled medication, joins an array of other DHE delivery systems, including an existing nasal spray, IV, and injectable forms. Levadex has proven its efficacy in treating acute migraine in phase III clinical trials, it has fewer side effects than triptans, overall, and it is as effective but more accessible than its IV counterpart.

Possible New Treatments for Other Common Headaches

There do not seem to be any "great, new breakthroughs" in medications used to treat tension-type headache (TTH). But I believe there is great promise in treating patients who experience frequent tension headaches or cervicogenic headaches with nondrug therapies, including acupuncture, biofeedback, myofascial release, and trigger point therapies.

Studies supported by the National Institute of Neurological Disorders and Stroke (NINDS), a part of the National Institutes of Health, are revealing new insights about headaches that may lead to innovative new treatments and additional avenues for blocking debilitating headache pain. I also believe that educating people who have headaches, as I have tried to do in this What Nurses Know guide, is a key to empowerment.

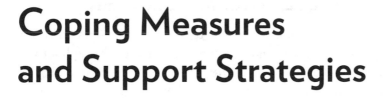

Coping Measures
and Support Strategies

*I've had headaches since I was a teenager, and I remember my
father having severe headaches, too, at the end of a hard day
at work. My son had headaches all through his school years,
and my grandson has now developed migraines at the age of
6. It's clear that headaches run in our family, and genetics are
not something any of us can change. But I try to stay in shape,
exercise, and avoid stress. I generally eat regular meals and
try to drink enough water. I've never smoked, and I rarely drink
alcohol. These are the only factors I can control in an attempt
to decrease the frequency of my headaches, and I try to pass
this lifestyle on to others in my family who get headaches. I
think of this as what I have to do to stay healthy, similar to
what my wife has to do to manage her Type 2 diabetes. In our
family, we support each other, which is a tremendous help to
all of us.* JAY

When headaches don't go away, developing coping tools is a necessity. Here you'll find information on gaining support from others who suffer from chronic headaches or other chronic pain. You'll learn how the Family Medical Leave Act (FMLA) can be used to help your family. The employer's role in accommodating employees with chronic headaches is discussed, important information for you to know if you want to keep your current position. Finally, you'll understand how to begin the application process for receiving disability benefits.

Finding Support in Your Community

Living with chronic headaches can be difficult for patients and their families. We've discussed many of these challenges throughout the book. What must it be like to meet with other people who know exactly what you're going through, who may be able to offer suggestions, names of physicians to contact, or simply offer to listen? I can tell you from first-hand experience, it's empowering! It's such a relief to have a safe place to unburden yourself—one place where you can be totally honest without fear of hurting someone's feelings: the doctor who you know has tried everything, the spouse who sometimes is unthinking or impatient. I'm talking about a support group for people with headaches or migraines specifically, or alternatively, a support group for people facing chronic pain.

Beyond the benefits of emotional support, local groups may bring in speakers with the latest information on new treatments and help to educate patients, spouses, and other family members. Some groups are involved in advocacy, working on legislative issues to include migraine in the list of disorders recognized by Social Security Disability, or campaigning for better funding for headache research. Other groups focus more exclusively on patient peer-support. While there may still be support groups in some communities, many groups now meet online and through social media websites.

The National Headache Foundation is the world's largest voluntary support organization for headache sufferers, and is a good source for locating information and support. See: www.headaches.org

The American Headache Society offers resources and support for headache patients as well as continuing education for health professionals through their education arm: ACHE–AHS Committee

What Nurses Know...

One recent study using 185 headache patients has shown that those who received peer-support from an interactive website, painACTION (www.painaction.com) had measurable improvements in categories such as:
- *Feeling empowered*
- *Use of relaxation strategies*
- *Use of social support*
- *Depression*
- *Ability to handle stress*

They were also less likely than headache patients who did not receive this support to "catastrophize" their pain, and in general, felt they were better able to cope with their pain. Using the painACTION website, patients who completed self-assessments of their coping skills and social interaction received immediate feedback and recommendations for improvement. It's important to note, however, that using the site did not alter pain levels—but assessments in coping with stress, feeling supported, and ability to handle pain increased significantly after one, three and six month intervals.

for Headache Education. See the following websites for more information:

www.americanheadachesociety.org
www.achenet.org

The American Academy of Neurology is one of the best sources of the latest information on advances in headache and migraine care, as well as information on related neurological disorders like epilepsy and traumatic brain injury. This organization also provides a wealth of education services for continuing medical education, helping physicians to stay on top of clinical practice guidelines.

See: www.aan.com

The American Migraine Foundation provides educational information for patients and health professionals and encourages greater awareness of migraine as a health disorder, including in schools. See the following website: www.americanmigrainefoundation.org

These organizations, and many others, also offer online forums and links to social media websites where patients can ask questions that those with more experience take the time to answer. See the *Resources* section for more information on headache support organizations.

Accommodating Chronic Headaches in the Workplace

When faced with a valuable employee who is experiencing distressing headaches, some employers are accommodating as much as possible, making more favorable changes in:

- Lighting
- Computer screen glare
- Relocating employees to quieter areas or reducing noise levels
- Enforcing fragrance- and smoke-free environments
- Educating supervisors about the employee's condition
- Offering flexible scheduling
- Allowing the possibility of telecommuting during headache periods

Not all people with migraines or other chronic headache conditions will need these accommodations, but making these changes may help to retain valuable and experienced employees. Migraineurs and others who suffer severe headache conditions should also take the initiative to screen for possible environmental triggers before accepting employment and should inform employers, supervisors, and, if appropriate, close-proximity coworkers about their health condition in advance of an attack or episode. If the work environment is deemed safe and the employer is accommodating, patients then need to make it a priority to be prepared for headaches that strike while on the job by bringing acute symptomatic medications to the workplace. For more ideas on accommodating employees with migraine and other headaches in the workplace, see: http://askjan.org/corner/vol02iss04.htm

How the Family Medical Leave Act Can Help Your Family

You may also want to consider whether you, your spouse, or other family may be eligible to take time off under the FMLA. Passed in 1993 with expected revisions in 2012, the FMLA allows eligible employees to take up to 12 weeks of unpaid leave off in any 12-month period for any of the following reasons:

- To help in the care or support of an employee's ill family member, including a spouse, minor child, or parent.
- To care for a newly born or newly adopted child, or a foster child who has recently been placed in an employee's care.
- The employee has an illness or health condition which makes it impossible to work.
- The employee must participate in National Guard or Reserve deployments or other related mandatory activities.
- The employee is responsible for caring for an active-duty Military service member who has suffered serious injury or illness. In this case, the employee may take a total of 26 weeks of leave in a 12-month period.

The FMLA protects employees from being dismissed, fired, or laid-off from their previous position due to a need to take time off related to the specific reasons listed above. You must be reinstated to the same or equivalent job upon your return and your employer must continue group health benefits while you are on leave. The FMLA can only be applied with medium-to-large companies employing more than 50 workers for at least 20 weeks of the current or preceding year. The employee requesting leave under the FMLA must have occupied his or her position for at least 12 months (not necessarily consecutive) and must have accrued 1,250 hours during the period of time immediately preceding the requested leave.

Employee responsibilities include requesting leave 30 days prior to beginning time off, or, in the event of unforeseen circumstances, requesting leave as soon as it is possible. An example of this would be receiving notice that a family member had been gravely injured and you needed to be available immediately, and for an extended period of time to follow.

Under the FMLA employees have the option of requesting a reduced work schedule, intermittent leave in specified blocks of time, or full-time leave. Persons requesting leave may be asked to present medical documentation of illness in themselves or a family member, but here the Health Insurance Portability and Accountability Act (HIPAA) law protects our privacy. Employers or supervisors may not contact health care providers directly, and health care providers may only provide information related to the health condition for which the employee is requesting leave.

Returning to the workplace also requires some planning and effort on the part of employees. They must inform the employer about the desire to return to work and the expected time-frame. If requested, the employee must also provide documentation that he or she is ready to return to work and will be able to carry out previous duties. Some individual states have family and medical leave laws. More information is available from your state's labor office.

Applying for Disability for Chronic Headaches

When headaches are out of control, the pain and other associated symptoms of migraine, cluster, and other severe headaches can make it impossible for a person to continue working. This may be a temporary situation until adequate treatment can be obtained, or, in some difficult-to-treat cases, disability may be long-term or permanent. Sometimes people are dealing with multiple health conditions at the same time, but often frequent headaches are "the straw that breaks the camel's back" and makes it impossible to continue to work. Navigating the maze of medical appointments and striving to live a normal home life are the bare necessities that can be managed. Some patients who are clearly struggling are reluctant to depend on governmental assistance. In the United States, we can be proud of the fact that our government has built-in safeguards to help its citizens in times of distress—and most of us have contributed financially to this system for our entire working lives by paying social security and income taxes. Migraine and cluster headache disorders are biologically-based neurological disorders and deserve to be treated like other biologically-based neurological disorders, even though the symptoms may not be outwardly visible to others. Sometimes we all need a little help.

In certain work environments, medical conditions like complicated migraine can make it unsafe, or even extremely dangerous to continue working in certain positions. If a migraineur suffers from temporary weakness or even paralysis, has sudden-onset visual defects associated with aura, dizziness or vertigo, or projectile vomiting, it may be simply impossible to continue one's work life. People who face months or years of intractable migraine or the various neuralgias face similar difficulties.

If you find yourself unable to continue working, you will need your physician's help to apply for social security disability. It's helpful to begin with an objective assessment focusing on your headache's impact on work routines and your ability to complete your assigned tasks. This can be accomplished in various ways, including using questionnaires like the Migraine Disability Assessment Questionnaire (MIDAS) or having patients complete simple online surveys available from the National Migraine Association or The American Council for Headache Education. Of course, the most significant evidence of the full impact of your health condition on your ability to work is your medical record, along with your doctor's physical and neurological assessment.

Using migraine as an example, the following information helps to explain how chronic and severe headache-related conditions are viewed in terms of disability:

The Americans with Disability Act (ADA) does not contain a list of medical conditions that constitute disabilities. Instead, the ADA has a general definition of disability that each person must meet. A person has a disability if he/she has a physical or mental impairment that substantially limits one or more major life activities, a record of such an impairment, or is regarded as having such an impairment. According to the Equal Employment Opportunity Commission (EEOC), having migraine headaches is an impairment. Therefore, people with migraine headaches who are substantially limited in a major life activity will have a disability under the ADA.

—JOB ACCOMMODATION NETWORK, A DIVISION OF THE OFFICE
OF DISABILITY EMPLOYMENT POLICY, U.S. DEPARTMENT OF
LABOR (2008)

Online headache patient forums can be helpful and encouraging when beginning the process of applying for disability, but someone else's experience may not be the same as *yours*. For the most accurate and up-to-date information, see the following resources:

"Social Security Disability Programs Can Help"—Online brochure from the Social Security Administration
"What You Need To Know When You Get Disability Benefits"—Online brochure from the Social Security Administration

In the United States, disability benefits are administered by the Social Security Administration (SSA), which oversees two programs: Social Security Disability and Supplemental Security Income (SSI). Disability qualifications may include the following:

- You have worked for the required period of time and earned a specific number of work credits.
- You are not able to work, or are working only marginally.
- It can be verified that your health condition interferes with work-related activities.
- Your condition appears on the SSA's list of disabling conditions (neither migraine nor headache do), or your condition is severe enough to prevent carrying out your previous work position.
- You are unable to adjust to other work offered by your employer (or your health condition prevents you from doing so). Usually you must be unable to perform almost all jobs, not just the job you were trained to do.
- Your disability has lasted or is expected to last at least 1 year or end in your death.

If you feel you meet the above criteria, and it can be verified by medical records provided by your physician, you may want to investigate the next steps to take in applying for disability by browsing the information on the SSA website's "Disability Planner": www.ssa.gov/dibplan/index.htm

The SSA also focuses more on the employee's inability to perform the job function than on specific diagnoses. So, even though migraine and other primary headache *aren't* specifically included in the SSA's list of accepted medical disabilities, disability benefits have been granted provided the condition is significantly "disabling."

The National Migraine Association (M.A.G.N.U.M.) and others are encouraging the addition of migraine criteria to Title II of the Americans with Disabilities Act (ADA). Some patients with chronic migraine have been able to qualify for disability, but application denial is not uncommon. It helps to be prepared to know you may be unsuccessful on your first attempt, and may need to appeal, possibly with the help of a disability attorney. How long the process takes depends in part on the demand in the area where you live. In some areas of the country, with large population sizes or heavy industry, it can, unfortunately, take quite a long time.

Additional Resources

The *Resources* section of the book offer additional sources of information on headache disorders, pain management, and support organizations. Please see also the Appendix, the sample headache diary, and the book's glossary. If you wish to contact me directly, you may do so through the book's publisher, Demos Health. I wish you the very best in health.

Glossary

Abdominal breathing: Drawing the breath deep into the abdomen so that the belly, not only the chest, rises, a technique commonly used in relaxation and yoga breathing.

Abortive (abortive medication): Used in this book to indicate a medication designed to alleviate or break a headache, as opposed to a medication used to prevent headaches; also referred to as a symptomatic medication.

Acute: Sudden onset, serious, or severe; an acute illness as opposed to a chronic illness.

Allergen: Any substance that triggers or induces an allergy attack including the release of histamine and other inflammatory substances.

Allodynia (cutaneous allodynia): Pain, irritation, or heightened sensitivity triggered by ordinary, nonpainful stimuli; associated with migraine headache and some other neurological disorders.

Amnesia: A temporary or permanent loss of memory for a given time period or event.

Analgesic: A pain relieving medication or effect.

Anecdotal: Based on personal or secondhand accounts rather than scientific investigation.

Aneurysm: A balloon-like sac formed by stretching of a weakened area of an artery or blood vessel; may rupture, causing catastrophic bleeding.

Anoxia: An absence of oxygen supply to an organ's tissues, leading to cellular death.

Antihistamine: A substance which helps to reduce the action of histamine, an inflammatory chemical produced in the body in response to injury or allergic reaction, by blocking the body's histamine receptors.

Aphasia: Difficulty speaking or understanding spoken and written language, usually due to injury to a specific speech-related area of the brain.

Arachnoid membrane: One of the three membranes that cover the brain; it lies between the pia mater and the dura. Collectively, these three membranes form the meninges.

Aura: Abnormal sensations and nervous system manifestations experienced prior to a migraine headache, and also prior to seizures in certain individuals; may involve visual disturbances, smelling unusual odors, tactile sensations, unusual tastes, or changes in hearing; these changes are temporary and usually transient—occurring for only a brief period of time.

Autoimmune disorder: Any disorder caused by the body's immune system attacking the body's own organs and tissues; autoimmune disorders include many common chronic health disorders and they are more frequently found in women.

AVM—arteriovenous malformation: An abnormal cluster of tangled blood vessels, arteries and veins in the brain which can contain weakened areas that rupture and bleed, causing neurological symptoms and possibly leading to loss of life.

Bilateral: Affecting or pertaining to both sides of the body.

Biofeedback: A method of helping a patient learn to control bodily functions not normally consciously controlled, using special sensors and a trained therapist; biofeedback can be used to learn to moderate the pain response.

Brain death: An irreversible stopping of measurable brain function; death.

CAM: A commonly used abbreviation for "Complementary and Alternative Medicine."

Celiac disease: A hereditary autoimmune disorder associated with the inability to digest proteins found in wheat, barley, rye, and related gluten-containing grains; celiac disease results in inflammation and can contribute to, or cause, headaches in certain individuals; the most critical treatment for celiac disease is a permanent lifelong avoidance of these gluten proteins.

Cephalgia: The technical medical term for headache; ceph- refers to head and -algia refers to pain.

Cerebrospinal fluid (CSF): The special fluid that bathes, cushions, and protects the brain and spinal cord.

Chronic (chronic condition): An illness or condition lasting over a long period of time, usually defined as longer than 3 to 6 months, which sometimes can be successfully managed, but not cured.

Closed head injury: An injury to the head in which the skull is not fractured; usually caused when the head violently strikes a hard surface.

Cognition: Referring to thought processes, memory, judgment, and other higher functions of the brain.

Coma: A state of profound unconsciousness and unresponsiveness caused by disease, injury, or metabolic changes in the body, including those caused by toxicity.

Comorbid: When illnesses, conditions, or disorders occur together, usually without a known or defined relationship.

Complementary medicine: A range of therapies addressing the cause and prevention of illness that lies outside the boundaries of conventional Western medicine; including nontraditional techniques such as acupuncture and herbal medicine.

Computed tomography (CT): A scan that creates a series of cross-sectional X-rays of the head and brain; also called computerized axial tomography or CAT scan.

Concussion: A mild to moderate injury to the brain, usually caused by a blow to the head or violent shaking motion, which can result in temporary confusion, disorientation, loss of memory, or short loss of consciousness.

Contagious; contagious illness: Illness spread by human contact or otherwise easily transmitted between those who have the condition and those in their immediate environment; the common cold is a contagious viral illness.

Contraceptive: A medication or device designed to prevent pregnancy.

Contrecoup: An area of swelling in the brain resulting from the shaking of the brain back and forth within the hard outer covering of the skull.

Contusion: A distinct area of swollen brain tissue including the presence of blood from broken blood vessels.

Cytokine: A group of chemicals produced by cells in the body that lead to inflammation.

Deep vein thrombosis (DVT): Formation of a blood clot deep within a vein (the blood vessels that carry blood back to the heart).

Depressed skull fracture: Fracture occurring when pieces of broken skull press into brain tissues.

Double-blind: Refers to studies in which the variables are unknown to both the study subject and the tester or researcher through use of special testing techniques; double-blind studies are respected as being unlikely to be influenced by researcher or participant bias.

Dura: A tough, fibrous membrane lining the brain; the outermost of the three membranes that collectively are called the meninges.

Dysarthria: Inability or difficulty articulating words due to emotional stress, brain injury, paralysis, or spasticity of the muscles needed for speech.

Epidural: Can refer to the anatomical epidural space, or in popular use, to epidural anesthesia given for surgical purposes or during labor.

Epidural hematoma: A pocket or area of heavy bleeding into the area between the skull and the dura, caused by damage to a major blood vessel within the cranium, or skull.

Episodic: Symptoms occurring in discrete "episodes," usually without a regular, predictable nature.

Fascia: Thin layer of fibrous connective tissue surrounding each of the organs of the body and also enclosing, binding together, and separating the muscle fibers and bundles.

Fatigue: Abnormal, dysfunctional feeling of weakness and lack of energy associated with many health conditions, including CFS–chronic fatigue syndrome.

Glasgow Coma Scale: A clinical tool used to assess the degree of consciousness and neurological functioning and reflecting the severity of brain injury–includes testing and ranking motor responsiveness, verbal acuity, and eye opening.

Global aphasia: A condition in which patients suffer severe communication disabilities as a result of extensive damage to portions of the brain responsible for language.

Guillain–Barré syndrome: A postviral neurological condition characterized by weakness and sometimes paralysis, often temporary.

Hemorrhagic stroke: A type of stroke caused by bleeding from one of the major arteries leading to the brain.

Holistic: Taking into account all of a person's physical, emotional, psychological, and social factors in the consideration and treatment of illness, health maintenance, and well-being.

Hyperacusis: An inability to tolerate sounds in the normal range; a form of increased sensitivity associated with migraine headache disorder.

Hypoxia: Decreased oxygen levels in an organ, such as the brain; less severe than anoxia.

Idiopathic: Occurring for reasons which are unknown.

Integrative: A practice of medicine utilizing or "integrating" traditional Western medicine with Holistic or Complementary medicine techniques, practiced by individuals or through an Integrative group medical practice.

Intracranial: Within the cranium, or skull or referring to locations within the brain.

Intracranial pressure: Buildup of pressure in the brain as a result of injury.

Intractable: Difficult to solve or manage successfully, as in an intractable condition.

Intravenous or IV medications: Medications given into the veins, usually by physicians, nurses, or other trained medical personnel.

Invasive: Referring to medical treatment involving insertion of something into a patient's body through a natural opening, a puncture in the skin, or a surgical incision.

Ischemic stroke: Stroke caused by the formation of a clot that blocks blood flow through an artery to the brain.

Lumbar puncture (also called a spinal tap): A sterile procedure done to obtain a sample of cerebrospinal fluid (CSF) by puncturing the spinal column at the base, below the level of the spinal cord.

Magnetic resonance imaging (MRI): A noninvasive diagnostic technique that uses magnetic fields to detect subtle changes in brain tissue.

Meningitis: Inflammation of the three membranes that envelop the brain and spinal cord, collectively known as the meninges; the meninges include the dura, pia mater, and arachnoid.

Migraineur: An individual who suffers from migraines.

Neuralgia: Constant or near-constant pain, tingling, or burning associated with chronic nerve irritation, usually limited to the nerve pathway, or distribution of the nerve's impulses.

Neuroexcitation: The electrical activation of cells in the brain; neuroexcitation is part of the normal functioning of the brain but can also be the result of abnormal activity related to an injury.

Neuron: A nerve cell; one of the main functional cells of the brain and nervous system.

Neuropathic pain: A type of pain caused by damage to or dysfunction in an area of the nervous system; can take many forms, including peripheral neuropathy affecting the extremities.

Neurotransmitters: Chemicals that transmit nerve signals from one neuron (nerve cell) to another.

NSAID: Nonsteroidal antiinflammatory drug; these include ibuprofen, naproxen, indomethacin, ketoprofin, aspirin, and many other over-the-counter and prescription medications.

Obesity: Severely overweight; the clinical definition of obesity is having a body mass index of 30 or higher; a cofactor in many health conditions.

Occipital: Referring to the back of the head, the occiput of the skull.

Off-label; off-label use: Refers to a use of a medication for another purpose than that for which the medication is approved.

OTC: An abbreviation for medications which can be purchased without a doctor's prescription "over the counter" in drugstores and grocery markets.

Pathogen: A microorganism that causes disease or infection.

Penetrating head injury: A brain injury in which an object pierces the skull and enters the brain tissue.

Peripheral nervous system: The part of the nervous system that lies outside of the brain and spinal cord.

Phonophobia: Abnormally increased sensitivity to sound, common in migraine and some other headache conditions.

Photophobia: Abnormally increased sensitivity to light, common in migraine and some other headache conditions.

Placebo: Substance or treatment that does not contain the therapeutic effect but which is not obvious to the person receiving it. Used in controlled clinical studies, and there may be some benefit due to suggestion, hence the name "placebo effect".

Plasticity: Ability of the brain to adapt to deficits and injury through growth, change, and acceptance of certain functions by alternate parts of the brain.

Postconcussion syndrome (PCS): A complex condition that may include headache after head injury, memory deficits, psychological changes, and often amnesia for the event that caused the concussion and the surrounding time period.

Postdrome; postdromal: Referring to the final phase of the four phases of migraine; prodomal symptoms may include fatigue, disorientation, and a feeling of mental fogginess.

Postpartum: The period after a woman gives birth; also postpartum.

Preeclampsia: The medical condition preeclampsia during pregnancy results in high blood pressure, persistent swelling and excretion of large amounts of protein in the urine. It can progress to a life-threatening condition including seizures.

Prenatal: The period of gestation prior to birth; occurring during that time period.

Prevalence: The number of cases of a disease or condition occurring in a given population and time period.

Primary headache: A headache which is not caused by another condition or disease.

Prodrome; prodromal: Referring to the initial phase of the four phases of migraine; referring to highly variable events or symptoms that develop up to several days prior to headache onset.

Prophylactic: A preventive strategy, practice, device, or medication; as in prophylactic medications which may prevent migraines or other headaches.

PTSD: Posttraumatic stress disorder; a physical and mental health disorder associated with suffering traumatic events and injuries; often linked to combat experience.

Rebound headache: Also called medication overuse headache; too frequent use of certain medications may lead to more frequent, more severe headaches, including chronic daily headache.

Riboflavin—vitamin B2: A vitamin important to the nervous system and sometimes used in headache prevention.

SCD—Spreading Cortical Depression: A process involving changes in the activity of specific brain cells preceding development of migraine and other severe headaches.

Secondary headache: A headache that is occurs in relation to or is "secondary" to another condition or disease process.

Sedentary: Referring to lack of movement, or lack of exercise and physical fitness; thought to be a cofactor in many health conditions.

Seizure: An episode of abnormal activity of nerve cells in the brain causing strange sensations, emotions, and behavior, or sometimes convulsions, muscle spasms, and loss of consciousness.

Shaken baby syndrome: A severe form of head injury that occurs when an infant or small child is shaken forcibly enough to cause the brain to bounce against the skull; the degree of brain damage depends on the extent and duration of the shaking.

Sporadic: Occurring only occasionally and usually without predictability.

SSRI: Selective serotonin reuptake inhibitor, a class of antidepressants that help to elevate mood by regulating the level of the neurotransmitter serotonin in the brain.

Status migrainosus: A specific episode of migraine lasting longer than 4 days, often up to a week or more, and requiring specific management strategies.

Stroke: A neurologic event caused by the disruption of blood flow to the brain, caused by a blockage (ischemic stroke) or by rupture of vessels and bleeding in the brain (hemorrhage).

Subdural hematoma: Bleeding confined to the area between the dura and the arachnoid membranes.

Systemic: Referring to having effects throughout the system, or body, as in systemic disease—a disease that has effects on more than one organ or body system

TCM—Traditional Chinese Medicine: A system of medicine dating back thousands of years to ancient China, and which makes use of specific herbal remedies, acupuncture and acupressure, massage, and moxibustion (the burning of herbs against the skin), among other practices; medical practitioners can obtain an education and certification in TCM, and often combine these techniques with other holistic, naturopathic, or allopathic practices to treat the whole patient.

Thrombosis or thrombus: The formation of a blood clot at the site of an injury.

TIA—Transient Ischemic Attack: Also called a ministroke, these small, temporary periods of reduced blood flow to the brain may be precursors to a more severe stroke; symptoms may overlap with, or be misdiagnosed as migraine, and vice versa.

Traumatic Brain Injury (TBI): Impairment of structures or functions of the brain resulting from traumatic injury, or repeated injury.

Tricyclic antidepressants: An older category of antidepressant medications, some of which are still used effectively to treat chronic pain.

Trigeminal nerve: One of the major branches of the cranial nerves providing nerve sensation and motor function to the head and face; the paired fifth cranial nerves.

Trigger (or headache trigger, specifically): A stimulus which sets off a biological process or leads to a migraine or other severe headache, including dietary, psychological, and environmental factors, but also medications and procedures.

Trigger point: A tight knot of muscle tissue that can often be felt by pressing firmly with the finger tips against a flat muscle; these sensitive points can radiate pain to other nearby areas of the body; there are various methods used to treat them, some of which you can learn to do yourself.

Triptans: A class of medications commonly used to treat migraine headaches, but also cluster headaches, and severe headaches from other disorders such as the autoimmune disorder lupus.

Unilateral: One-sided, or referring to one side of the body.

Vasoconstriction: When blood vessels narrow, constricting the flow of blood.

Vasodilation: When blood vessels dilate or widen, expanding the flow of blood.

Vasospasm: Exaggerated, persistent contraction of the walls of a blood vessel.

Vertigo: An abnormal spinning sensation of acute dizziness accompanied by nausea and vomiting and a feeling that one's surroundings are revolving.

Vesicles: Small, fluid-filled blisters erupting on the skin, associated with the disorder known as shingles, caused by the herpes zoster virus.

Viral meningitis: A viral illness causing inflammation and irritation of the meninges surrounding the brain, causing severe pain, nausea, sensitivity to light and sound, and other symptoms.

Visualization: The process of consciously creating a vivid mental picture of a thing, place, or positive outcome in order to gain a greater sense of well-being or reach a desired mental state.

Resources for Headache Patients

Organizations and Contact Information

American Academy of Neurology
www.aan.com
800.879.1960 or 651.695.2717
Fax: 651.695.2791
Email: memberservices@aan.com

American Council for Headache Education (ACHE)
www.achenet.org
This organization offers support groups throughout the country.
856.423.0043
Fax: 856.423.0082
Email: achehq@talley.com

American Headache Society
The American Headache Society offers resources and support for headache patients, as well as continuing education for health professionals through their education arm: ACHE–AHS Committee for Headache Education. See the following website for more information: www.americanhead achesociety.org/support

American Migraine Foundation
www.americanmigrainefoundation.org

American Pain Foundation
www.painfoundation.org
888.615.7246
Email: info@painfoundation.org

I hate headches.org patient support website
www.ihateheadaches.org/headache-support-groups.html

National Center for Complementary and Alternative Medicine
www.nccam.nih.gov
888.644.6226/Fax: 866.464.3616
Email: info@nccam.nih.gov

National Headache Foundation
www.headaches.org
(888) NHF-5552 or 312.274.2650
Fax: 773.525.7357
Email: info@headaches.org

The National Headache Foundation is the world's largest voluntary support organization for headache sufferers and is a good source for locating groups in 23 U.S. states. See: www.headaches.org/NHF_Programs/
Support_Groups

National Institutes of Health (NIH)
National Institute of Neurological Disorders and Stroke
NIH Neurological Institute
301.496.5751 or 800.352.9424
www.ninds.nih.gov

PainAction.com interactive website
www.painaction.com
One study showed that participants had measurable improvements in coping ability with its use.

For further information and reading on headaches, see the Bibliography.

Bibliography

Introduction

"Epidemiology and Impact of Headache and Migraine." http://www.american-headachesociety.org/assets/1/7/NAP_for_Web_-_Epidemiology__Impact_of_Headache__Migraine.pdf

Hawkins, K., S. Wang, and M. Rupnow. "Indirect Cost Burden of Migraine in the United States." *Journal of Occupational & Environmental Medicine* 49, no. 4 (2007): 368–74.

Lipton, R., M. Bigal, M. Diamond, F. Freitag, M.L. Reed, W.F. Stewart, and on behalf of the AMPP Advisory Group. "Migraine Prevalence, Disease Burden, and the Need for Preventive Therapy." *Neurology* 68, no. 5 (2007): 343–9.

MacGregor, E., J. Brandes, and A. Eikermann. "The Migraine and Zolmitriptan Evaluation (MAZE) Study." In *Study presented at the American Academy of Neurology 2001 Annual Meeting*, Philadelphia, May 5–11, 2001.

Medstat, Thomson. "New Data Estimate Migraine Headaches Cost U.S. Employers More Than $24 Billion Annually." http://www.prnewswire.com/news-releases/new-data-estimate-migraine-headaches-cost-us-employers-more-than-24-billion-annually-56974912.html

National Headache Foundation. "National Headache Foundation Fact Sheet." http://www.health-exchange.net/pdfdb/headfactEng.pdf

Stovner, L., K. Hagen, R. Jensen, Z. Katsarava, R. Lipton, A. Scher, T. Steiner, and J.A. Zwart. The Global Burden of Headache: A Documentation of Headache Prevalence and Disability Worldwide. *Cephalalgia* 27 (2007): 193–210.

University of Maryland Medical Center. "Tension Headache Described." http://www.umm.edu/altmed/articles/tension-headache-000074.htm

Wang, Y., J. Zhou, X. Fan, X. Li, L. Ran, G. Tan, L. Chen, K. Wang, and B. Liu. "Classification and Clinical Features of Headache Patients: An Outpatient Clinic Study From China." *Journal of Headache Pain* 12, no. 5 (2011): 561–7.

Chapter 1: Headache Basics—Living With Problem Headaches

Bigal, M., and J. Gladstone. "The Metabolic Headaches." *Current Pain and Headache Report* 12, no. 4 (2008): 292–5. http://www.ncbi.nlm.nih.gov/pubmed/18625107.

Burstein, R., D. Yarnitsky, I. Goor-Aryeh, B. Ransil, and Z. Bajwa. "An Association Between Migraine and Cutaneous Allodynia." *Annals of Neurology* 47, no. 5 (2000): 614–24.

Childers, L. "Cindy's Campaign." *Neurology Now* 6, no. 3 (2010): 16–9.

Cutrer, M., and M. Moskowitz. "Headaches and Other Head Pain: Pathophysiology." http://www.healthline.com/elseviercontent/cecil-headaches-and-other-head-pain/2#ixzz1KP7RVAUO

Didion, Joan. "In Bed" from *The White Album*. New York: Simon & Schuster, 1979.

Dodick, D. "Diagnosing Headache: Clinical Clues and Clinical Rules." *Advanced Studies in Medicine* 3, no. 2 (2003): 87–92. http://www.jhasim.com/files/articlefiles/pdf/journal_p87(V3-2)AmbulatoryM.pdf.

GlaxoSmithKline. "The Headache Impact Test—How Much Are Headaches Disrupting Your Life?" http://www.headachetest.com/

Headache Classification Subcommittee of the International Headache Society. http://ihs-classification.org/en/

James, Frank. "Michele Bachmann's Migraines are Latest Question About Rising Political Star." 2011. http://www.npr.org/blogs/itsallpolitics/2011/07/19/138519042/michele-bachmanns-migraines-are-latest-question-about-rising-political-star

Kamen, P. *All in My Head: An Epic Quest to Cure an Unrelenting, Totally Unreasonable, and Only Slightly Enlightening Headache.* Cambridge, MA: Da Capo Press, 2006.

Marcus, D. *Headache and Chronic Pain Syndromes: The Case-Based Guide to Targeted Assessment and Treatment.* Totowa, NJ: Humana Press, 2007.

MigraineInformation.org. "Headache Statistics." http://www.migraineinfor mation.org/migraine-help/headache-statistics.htm

National Institute of Neurological Disorders and Stroke. "Headache: Hope Through Research." http://www.ninds.nih.gov/disorders/headache/detail_ headache.htm

Pryse-Phillips, W., and T. Murray. "Mechanisms of Cranial Pain, in Headaches and Other Head Pain." In *Textbook of Primary Care Medicine.* 3rd ed. http://www.healthline.com/elseviercontent/textbook-headache/2#ixzz1KP8UkrKG

Chapter 2: Understanding Risk Factors and Headache Triggers

Bauer, A. "Vitamin D and Migraine Headaches." 2010. http://www.livestrong. com/article/274585-vitamin-d-and-migraine-headaches/

Bigal, M., A. Tsang, E. Loder, D. Serrano, M.L. Reed, and R.B. Lipton. "Body Mass Index and Episodic Headaches: A Population-Based Study." *Archives of Internal Medicine* 167, no. 18 (2007): 1964-70.

Cassels, Caroline. "Vitamin D Deficiency Common in Patients with Chronic Migraine." In *American Headache Society 50th Annual Scientific Meeting: Abstract S33.* 2008. http://www.medscape.com/viewarticle/577151

Cathcart, S., J. Petkov, A. Winefield, K. Lushington, and P. Rolan. "Central Mechanisms of Stress-Induced Headache." *Cephalalgia* 30, no. 3 (2009): 285-95.

Centers for Disease Control and Prevention. "Facts About Stachybotrys char-tarum and Other Molds." http://www.cdc.gov/mold/stachy.htm

Centers for Disease Control and Prevention. "Sleep and Sleep Disorders." http://www.cdc.gov/Features/Sleep/

Cigna. "Headache Triggers." http://www.cignabehavioral.com/web/basicsite/ bulletinBoard/headacheTriggers.jsp

Cowan, R., and S. Sahai. "Causes and Treatments of Migraine and Related Headaches." http://www.emedicinehealth.com/causes_and_treatments_of_ migraine_headaches/article_em.htm

Cunha, J. "Jet Lag." Medicinet. http://www.medicinenet.com/jet_lag/article.htm

Cynthia Peterson. "The TMJ Healing Plan: Ten Steps to Relieving Persistent Jaw, Neck and Head Pain." Alameda, CA: Hunter House, 2010.

Gandey, A. "Vitamin D Low in Patients With Headache and Migraine." In *American Headache Society (AHS) 52nd Annual Scientific Meeting: Poster 51.* 2010. http://www.medscape.com/viewarticle/724646

Gordon, D., R. Hamel, and A. Lake. *Non-Drug Treatment Alternatives.* Michigan Headache Institute. http://www.mhni.com/faqs_non_drug.aspx

Kirk, R. "30 Possible Migraine and Headache Triggers." http://www.backinac tion.net/article-migrainetrigger.html

Levine, B. *Your Body Needs Water!* By Linda Heywood. Bella Online. Linda Heywood Bella Online's Holistic Health Editor Your Body Needs Water!

LeWine, H. *Ask the Expert: Can Dehydration Cause Headaches?* Aetna Intellihealth, 2009. http://www.intelihealth.com/IH/ihtIH/WSIHW000/ 4464/8480/465540.html

Lyngberg, A., B. Rasmussen, T. Jørgensen, and R. Jensen. "Incidence of Primary Headache: A Danish Epidemiologic Follow-up Study." *American Journal of Epidemiology* 161, no. 11 (2005): 1066–73.

Marsili, S., and M. Pontell. "Anatomical Connection Between the Rectus Capitis Posterior Major and the Dura Mater." *Spine* 36, no. 25 (2011): E1612–4.

Michigan Headache & Neurological Institute. "Non-Drug Treatment Alternatives." http://www.mhni.com/faqs_non_drug.aspx#Diet

Mukamal, K., G. Wellenius, H. Suh, and M. Mittleman. "Weather and Air Pollution as Triggers of Severe Headaches." 72, no. 10 (2009): 922–7. http:// www.ncbi.nlm.nih.gov/pubmed/19273827

National Institute of General Medical Sciences. "Circadian Rhythms Fact Sheet." 2008. http://www.nigms.nih.gov/Education/Factsheet_ CircadianRhythms.htm

Ødegård, S., T. Sand, M. Engstrøm, L.J. Stovner, J.A. Zwart, and K. Hagen. "The Long-Term Effect of Insomnia on Primary Headaches: Discussion." *Headache* 51, no. 4 (2011): 570–80.

Paul, C., R. Au, L. Fredman, J.M. Massaro, S. Seshadri, C. Decarli, and P.A. Wolf. "Association of Alcohol Consumption with Brain Volume in the Framingham Study." *Archives of Neurology* 65, no. 10 (2008): 1363–67.

Peterson, C. "Obesity and Headache." http://www.migrainesurvival.com/ obesity

Robberstad, L., G. Dyb, K. Hagen, L.J. Stovner, T.L. Holmen, J.-A. Zwart. "An Unfavorable Lifestyle and Recurrent Headaches Among Adolescents. The HUNT Study." *Neurology* 75, no. 8 (2010): 712–7.

Sherris, D., E. Kern, and J. Ponikau. "Mayo Clinic Study Implicates Fungus as Cause of Chronic Sinusitis." 1999. http://www.princeton.edu/~gpmenos/ mold_facts/MayoClinicStudyImplicatesFungusasCauseofChronicSinusi.pdf

Stovner, L., K. Hagen, R. Jensen, Z. Katsarava, R. Lipton, A. Scher, T. Steiner, and J.A. Zwart. "The Global Burden of Headache: A Documentation of Headache Prevalence and Disability Worldwide." *Cephalalgia no.* 3 (2007): 193–210.

The Mayo Clinic Staff. "Migraine: Risk Factors." http://www.mayoclinic.com/ health/migraine-headache/DS00120/DSECTION=risk-factors

The University of Maryland Medical Center. "Headaches—Tension—Causes." http://www.umm.edu/patiented/articles/what_causes_tension_other_ chronic_daily_headaches_000011_3.htm

WebMD.com. "Sleep and Circadian Rhythm Disorders." 2010. http://www. webmd.com/sleep-disorders/guide/circadian-rhythm-disorders-cause

Wheeler, S., B. Gang, and F. Taylor. "Vitamin D, Migraine, and Health– Medical Complications: Optimize Therapy!" ACHE. http://www.achenet. org/resources/vitamin_d_migraine_and_health/

Young, W., and S. Silberstein. *Migraine and Other Headaches*. Demos Medical Publishing, 2004.

Chapter 3: A Headache Prevention Diet

Alpay, K., M. Ertas, K. Orhan, D.K. Ustay, C. Lieners, and B. Baykan. "Diet Restriction in Migraine, Based on IgG Against Foods: A Clinical Double-Blind, Randomised, Cross-Over Trial." *Cephalalgia* 30, no. 7 (2010): 829-37. http://www.ncbi.nlm.nih.gov/pmc/articles/PMC2899772/

Brainard, J. "Angiotensin and Aldosterone Elevation in Salt-Induced Migraine." *Headache: The Journal of Head and Face Pain* 21, no. 5 (1981): 222-26. http://onlinelibrary.wiley.com/doi/10.1111/j.1526-4610.1981.hed2105222.x/ abstract

D'Andrea, G., F. Granella, M. Leone, F. Perini, A. Farruggio, G. Bussone. "Abnormal Platelet Trace Amine Profiles in Migraine With and Without Aura." *Cephalalgia* 26, no. 8 (2006): 968-72. http://www.ncbi.nlm.nih.gov/ pubmed/16886933

D'Andrea, G., G. Nordera, F. Perini, G. Allais, and F. Granella. "Biochemistry of Neuromodulation in Primary Headaches: Focus on Anomalies of Tyrosine Metabolism." *Neurological Sciences* 28, Suppl. 2 (2007): S94-6. http://www. ncbi.nlm.nih.gov/pubmed/17508188

Egger, J., J. Wilson, C. Carter, M.W. Turner, and J.F. Soothill. "Is Migraine Food Allergy? A Double-Blind Controlled Trial of Oligoantigenic Diet Treatment." *Lancet* 2 (1983): 865-9. http://www.ncbi.nlm.nih.gov/ pubmed/6137694.

Gabey, A. "Migraine Headache–Nutrional Treatments. Dietary Factors." http://heartspring.net/migraine_headache_natural_treatments.html

George, D. "How Does Salt Cause Migraine Headaches?" http://www.ehow.com/ how-does_5003500_salt-cause-migraine-headaches.html#ixzz1nWOzCT4u

Grant, E. "Food Allergies and Migraine." *Lancet* 1 (1979): 966-9. http://www. ncbi.nlm.nih.gov/pubmed/87628.

Gupta, R., E. Springston, M. Warrier, B. Smith, R. Kumar, J. Pongracic, and J.L. Holl. "The Prevalence, Severity, and Distribution of Childhood Food Allergy in the United States." *Pediatrics*, 2011. http://pediatrics.aappubli-cations.org/content/early/2011/06/16/peds.2011-0204.abstract.

Healey, J. "A Lesser Known Migraine Trigger." 2008. http://health.ezine9. com/a-lesser-known-migraine-trigger-13ea58e288.html

Kaslow, J. *Health Topics* discussion of common triggers of food-related headaches. 2011. http://www.drkaslow.com/html/headaches_allergies___foods.html

Lionetti, E., R. Francavilla, L. Maiuri, M. Ruggieri, M. Spina, P. Pavone, T. Francavilla, A.M. Magistà, and L. Pavone. "Headache in Pediatric Patients with Celiac Disease and its Prevalence as a Diagnostic Clue." *Journal of Pediatric Gastroenterology and Nutrition* 49, no. 2 (2009): 202-7. http://www.ncbi.nlm.nih.gov/pubmed/19543115.

Lipton, R., L. Newman, J. Cohen, and S. Solomon. "Aspartame as a Dietary Trigger of Headache." *Headache* 29, no. 2: 90-2. http://www.ncbi.nlm.nih.gov/pubmed/2708042

Mcculloch, J., and A. Harper. "Phenylethylamine and Cerebral Blood Flow: Possible Involvement of Phenylethylamine in Migraine." *Neurology* 27, no. 9 (1977): 817-21. http://www.ncbi.nlm.nih.gov/pubmed/408734

Monro, J., C. Carini, and J. Brostoff. "Migraine is a Food Allergic Disease." *Lancet* 2 (1984): 719-21.

Patel, R., R. Sarma, and E. Grimsley. "Popular Sweetener Sucralose as a Migraine Trigger." *Headache* 46, no. 8 (2006): 1303-4. http://www.ncbi.nlm.nih.gov/pubmed/16942478

Paul, C., R. Au, L. Fredman, J. Massaro, S. Seshadri, C. Decarli, and P.A. Wolf. "Association of Alcohol Consumption with Brain Volume in the Framingham Study." *Archives of Neurology* 65, no. 10 (2008): 1363-67. http://www.ncbi.nlm.nih.gov/pmc/articles/PMC2861346/

Rubio-Tapia, A., R. Kyle, E.L. Kaplan, et al. "Increased Prevalence and Mortality in Undiagnosed Celiac Disease." *Mayo Gastroenterology* 137, no. 1 (2009): 88-93.

Sapers, G. "Browning of Foods: Control by Sulfites, Antioxidants, and Other Means." *Food Technology* 47, no. 10 (1993): 75-84.

Taylor, S., N. Higley, and R. Bush. "Sulfites in Foods: Uses, Analytical Lmethods, Redisues, Fate, Exposure Assessment, Metabolism, Toxicity, and Hypersensitivity." *Advances in Food Research* 30 (1986): 1-76.

Veracity, D. "Aspartame Consumption Strongly Associated with Migraines and Seizures." 2005. http://www.naturalnews.com/008797.html

Chapter 4: Finding Help for Your Headaches

Canter, L. "Anaphylactoid Reactions to Radiocontrast Media." *Allergy and Asthma Proceedings* 26 (2005): 199-203.

Detsky, M., D. McDonald, M. Baerlocher, G.A. Tomlinson, D.C. McCrory, and C.M. Booth. "Does This Patient with Headache Have a Migraine or Need Neuroimaging?" *Journal of the American Medical Association* 296 (2006): 1274-83.

Edlow, J., P. Panagos, S. Godwin, T. Thomas, and W. Decker. "Clinical Policy: Critical Issues in the Evaluation and Management of Adult Patients Presenting to the Emergency Department With Acute Headache." *Annals of Emergency Medicine* 52, no. 4 (2008): 407-36.

Kamen, P. *All in My Head: An Epic Quest to Cure an Unrelenting, Totally Unreasonable, and Only Slightly Enlightening Headache.* Cambridge, MA: Da Capo Press, 2006.

Kathula S, J. Mantil, T. Drehmer, and S. Patil. "Giant Cell Arteritis Mimicking Multiple Myeloma; Diagnosed by PET Scan." *Southern Medical Journal* 99, no. 11 (2006): 1280-81. http://www.medscape.com/viewarticle/549295

Lieberman, P., S.F. Kemp, J. Oppenheimer, et al. "The Diagnosis and Management of Anaphylaxis: An Updated Practice Parameter." *Journal of Allergy and Clinical Immunology* 115 (2005): S483-523.

More, D. *Iodine Contrast Allergy.* About.com Guide, 2009. http://allergies.about.com/od/medicationallergies/a/rcmallergy.htm

National Headache Foundation. "PET Scan." http://www.headaches.org/education/Headache_Topic_Sheets/PET_Scan

Neff, M. "Evidence-Based Guidelines for Neuroimaging in Patients with Nonacute Headache." *American Family Physician* 71, no. 6 (2005): 1219-22. http://www.aafp.org/afp/2005/0315/p1219.html.

Paula Ford-Martin. "Neuroimaging." http://www.netplaces.com/migraines/diagnosis/neuroimaging.htm

Pryse-Phillips, W., and J. Murray. *Headache.* Healthline.com, 1992. http://www.healthline.com/elseviercontent/textbook-headache/5#ixzz1KP8tVQvQ.

Pryse-Phillips, W., D. Dodick, J. Edmeads, M.J. Gawel, R.F. Nelson, R A. Purdy, G. Robinson, D. Stirling, and I. Worthington. "Guidelines for the Diagnosis and Management of Migraine in Clinical Practice." *Canadian Medical Association Journal* 156 (1997): 1273-8. http://www.cmaj.ca/content/156/9/1273.full.pdf

Radiologyinfo.org. "CT." http://www.radiologyinfo.org/en/info.cfm?pg=bodyct

The National Institute of Neurological Disorders and Stroke. "Headaches: Hope through Research." http://www.ninds.nih.gov/disorders/headache/detail_headache.htm

Universalium. "Nervous System Disease." http://universalium.academic.ru/280805/nervous_system_disease

Chapter 5: A Review of Complementary and Alternative Therapies

American Massage Therapy Associaton. "2011 Position Statement Proposal: Tension Headaches." http://www.amtamassage.org/positionintro/

2011-Position-Statement-Proposals/2011-Position-Statement-Proposal–Tension-Headaches0.html

Anderson, P. "Feverfew-Ginger Combo Safe, Effective in Treating Migraines." *Medscape Medical News*, 2011. http://www.medscape.com/viewarticle/745248

Assendelft, W., S. Morton, E. Yu, M.J. Suttorp, and P.G. Shekelle. "Spinal Manipulative Therapy for Low-Back Pain." *Annals of Internal Medicine* 138, no. 11 (2003): 871–81. http://www.annals.org/content/138/11/871.abstract

Bakalar, N. "Regimens: Acupuncture Provides Headache Relief." *The New York Times*, December 15, 2008. http://www.nytimes.com/2008/12/16/health/research/16regi.html

Blakeway, J. "Acupuncture for Headaches–Promising New Research." The YinOva Center. Traditional wisdom for Modern Families. http://www.yinovacenter.com/blog/archives/1009/.

Blatman, H. "How does Myofascial Pain Cause Headache? in Headache Pain Relief–Migraine Treatment: Frequently Asked Questions." http://www.blatmanpainclinic.com/Headache-and-Myofascial-Pain.htm

Cohen, A., B. Burns, and P. Goadsby. "High-Flow Oxygen for Treatment of Cluster Headache." *Journal of the American Medical Association* 302, no. 22 (2009): 2451–57.

Di Rosa, G., S. Attina, M. Spano, G. Ingegneri, D.L. Sgrò, G. Pustorino, M. Bonsignore, V. Trapani-Lombardo, and G. Tortorella. "Efficacy of Folic Acid in Children with Migraine, Hyperhomocysteinemi A and MTHFR Polymorphisms." *Headache* 47 (2007): 1342–44.

Diener, H., V. Pfaffenrath, J. Schnitker, M. Friede, and Z. Henneicke-von. "Efficacy and Safety of 6.25 Mg T.I.D. Feverfew CO2-Extract (MIG-99) in Migraine Prevention–A Randomized, Double-Blind, Multicentre, Placebo-Controlled Study." *Cephalalgia* 25, no. 11 (2005): 1031–41. http://www.ncbi.nlm.nih.gov/pubmed/16232154

Eggers, J. "Demystifying Myofascial Release." 2008. http://www.thedailyheadache.com/2008/03/understanding-fascia-and-myofascial-release.html

Facchinetti, F., G. Sances, P. Borella, A.R. Genazzani, and G. Nappi. "Magnesium Prophylaxis of Menstrual Migraine: Effects on Intracellular Magnesium." *Headache* 31 (1991): 298–304.

Gaby, A. "Riboflavin Relieves Migraine Headaches." Healthstatus.com. http://www.healthstatus.com/articles1/riboflavin-relieves-migraine-headaches/

Glueck, C., T. McCarren, R. Hitzemann, et al. "Amelioration of Severe Migraine with Omega-3 Fatty Acids: A Double-Blind, Placebo-Controlled Clinical Trial." *American Journal of Clinical Nutrition* 43 (1986): 710.

Grossman, P., L. Niemann, S. Schmidt, and H. Walach. "Mindfulness-Based Stress Reduction and Health Benefits. A Meta-Analysis." *Journal of*

Psychosomatic Research 57, no. 1 (2004): 35-43. http://www.ncbi.nlm.nih. gov/pubmed/15256293

Harel, Z., G. Gascon, S. Riggs, R. Vaz, W. Brown, and G. Exil. "Supplementation with Omega-3 Poly- Unsaturated Fatty Acids in the Management of Recurrent Migraines in Adolescents." *Journal of Adolescent Health* 31 (2002): 154-61.

Hershey, A., S. Powers, A. Vockell, S.L. Lecates, P.L. Ellinor, A. Segers, D. Burdine, P. Manning, and M.A. Kabbouche. "Coenzyme Q10 Deficiency and Response to Supplementation in Pediatric and Adolescent Migraine." *Headache* 47 (2007): 73-80.

Integrative Manual Therapy Association. "What is Integrative Manual Therapy?" http://www.imtassociation.org/what-is-imt.asp

Kaushik, R., R.M. Kaushik, S. Mahajan, and V. Rajesh. "Biofeedback Assisted Diaphragmatic Breathing and Systematic Relaxation Versus Propranolol in Long Term Prophylaxis of Migraine." *Complementary Therapies in Medicine* 13, no. 3 (2005): 165-74. http://www.ncbi.nlm.nih.gov/pubmed/16150370

Kerns, M. "Black Cohosh for Headaches." 2010. http://www.livestrong.com/ article/291513-black-cohosh-for-headaches/

Kiefer, D., and T. Pantuso. "Dietary Supplements Can be a Useful Part of an Integrative Approach to the Treatment of Pain." *Headache* 51, no. 3 (2011): 469-83.

Linde, K., G. Allais, B. Brinkhaus, E. Manheimer, A. Vickers, and A. White. "Acupuncture for Migraine Prophylaxis." *Cochrane Database System Review* no. 1 (2009): CD001218. http://www.ncbi.nlm.nih.gov/ pubmed/19160193

Maizels, M., A. Blumenfeld, and R. Burchette. "A Combination of Riboflavin, Magnesium, and Fever Few for Migraine Prophylaxis: A Randomized Trial." *Headache* 44 (2004): 885-90.

Maj, S. "New Study Shows How Chiropractic Can Help With Tension Headaches." 2011. http://drmaj.com/new-study-shows-how-chiropractic-can-help-with-tension-headaches/

Mayo Clinic Staff. "Alternative Medicine." http://www.mayoclinic.com/ health/migraine-headache/DS00120/DSECTION=alternative-medicine

Mayo Clinic Staff. "Black Cohosh (*Cimicifuga racemosa* [L.] Nutt.)." http:// www.mayoclinic.com/health/black-cohosh/NS_patient-blackcohosh

McCarren, T., R. Hitzemann, R. Smith, et al. "Amelioration of Severe Migraine by Fish Oil Omega-3 Fatty Acids." *American Journal of Clinical Nutrition* 41 (1985): 874.

Melchart, D., W. Weidenhammer, A. Streng, A. Hoppe, V. Pfaffenrath, and K. Linde. "Acupuncture for Chronic Headaches—An Epidemiological Study: Conclusion." *Headache* 46, no. 4 (2006): 632-41. http://www.medscape. com/viewarticle/530485_5

Michigan Headache and Neurological Institute. "Are There Non-Drug Alternatives?" http://www.mhni.com/faqs_non_drug.aspx

Narin, S., L. Pinar, E. Erbas, V. Oztürk, and F. Idiman. "The Effects of Exercise and Exercise-Related Changes in Blood Nitric Oxide Level on Migraine Headache." *Clinical Rehabilitation* 17, no. 6 (2003): 624-30. http://www.ncbi.nlm.nih.gov/pubmed/12971707

National College of Naturopathic Medicine. "Naturopathic Principles of Healing." http://www.ncnm.edu/academic-programs/school-of-naturopathic-medicine/about-naturopathic-medicine.php

Office of Dietary Supplements—National Institute of Health. "Dietary Supplement Fact Sheets." http://ods.od.nih.gov/factsheets/list-all/

Office of Dietary Supplements—National Institute of Health. "Dietary Supplement Fact Sheet: Black Cohosh." http://ods.od.nih.gov/factsheets/BlackCohosh-HealthProfessional/

Peikert, A., C. Wilimzig, and R. Kohne-Volland. "Prophylaxis of Migraine with Oral Magnesium: Results from a Prospective, Multi-Center, Placebo-Controlled and Double-Blind Randomized Study." *Cephalalgia* 16 (1996): 257-63.

Peterson, C. *Chapter 10—Halt Head and Neck Pain in the TMJ Healing Plan.* Alameda, CA: Hunter House Publishers, 2010.

Peterson, C. "Herbal Supplements and Medications: an Overview of Herb-Herb and Drug-Herb Interactions." Migraine Survival. http://www.migraine-survival.com/herbal-supplements-and-medications-an-overview-of-herb-herb-and-drug-herb-interactions

Quinn, C., C. Chandler, and A. Moraska. "Massage Therapy and Frequency of Chronic Tension Headaches." *American Journal of Public Health* 92, no. 10 (2002): 1657-61. http://www.ncbi.nlm.nih.gov/pmc/articles/PMC1447303/

Rozen, T., M. Oshinsky, C. Gebeline, K.C. Bradley, W.B. Young, A.L. Shechter, and S.D. Silberstein. "Open Label Trial of Coenzyme Q10 as a Migraine Preventive." *Cephalalgia* 22 (2002): 137-41.

Sandor, P., L. Di Clemente, G. Coppola, U. Saenger, A. Fumal, D. Magis, L. Seidel, R.M. Agosti, and J. Schoenen. "Efficacy of Coenzyme Q10 in Migraine Prophylaxis: A Randomized Controlled Trial." *Neurology* 64 (2005): 713-5.

Scali, F., E. Marsili, and M. Pontell. "Anatomical Connection Between the Rectus Capitis Posterior Major and the Dura Mater." *Spine* 36, no. 25 (2011): E1612-4. http://www.ncbi.nlm.nih.gov/pubmed/21278628

Schoenen, J., M. Lenaerts, and E. Bastings. "High-Dose Riboflavin as a Prophylactic Treatment of Migraine: Results of an Open Pilot Study." *Cephalalgia* 14 (1994): 328-9.

Soriani, S., C. Arnaldi, L. De Carlo, D. Arcudi, D. Mazzotta, P.A. Battistella, S. Sartori, and V. Abbasciano. "Serum and Red Blood Cell Magnesium Levels in Juvenile Migraine Patients." *Headache* 35 (1995): 14-6.

Stark, S. "Why Not Suggest Myofascial Therapy for Migraine?" Ask Dr. Stuart Stark. Everyday Health–Headache and Migraine. http://www.every dayhealth.com/headache-and-migraines/specialists/why-not-suggest-myofascial-therapy-for-migraine.aspx

Sun-Edelstein, C., and A. Mauskop. "Nutraceuticals, Behavioral and Physical Headache Treatments: Conclusions." *Headache* 51, no. 3 (2011): 469-83. http://www.medscape.com/viewarticle/738530_5

Tufts Medical Center. "Butterbur–*Petasites hybridus*." http://www.tufts-nemc.org/apps/HealthGate/Article.aspx?chunkiid=21626

Upledger Institute International. "Frequently Asked Questions–CranioSacral Therapy." http://www.upledger.com/content.asp?id=61

US Food and Drug Administration. "MedWatch: The FDA Safety Information and Adverse Event Reporting Program." www.fda.gov/medwatch/

Zhao, Stillman, Rozen. "Traditional and Evidence-Based Acupuncture in Headache: Conclusion." *Headache* 45, no. 6 (2005): 716-30. http://www.medscape.com/viewarticle/507374_7

Chapter 6: Tension-Type Headache

Bendtsen, L., and R. Jensen. "Tension-Type Headache." *Neurologic Clinics* 27, no. 2 (2009): 525-35.

Cutrer, Michael, and M. Moskowitz. "Headaches and Other Head Pain." From Healthline.com–Connect to Better Health. http://www.healthline.com/elseviercontent/cecil-headaches-and-other-head-pain/3#ixzz1KP7b1sj4

Foster, K.A., J. Liskin, S. Cen, A. Abbott, V. Armisen, D. Globe, L. Knox, M. Mitchell, C. Shtir, and S. Azen. "The Trager Approach in the Treatment of Chronic Headache: A Pilot Study." *Alternative Therapies in Health and Medicine* 10, no. 5 (2004): 40-6.

Gobel, H., V. Hamouz, C. Hansen, K. Heininger, S. Hirsch, V. Lindner, D. Heuss, and D. Soyka. "Chronic Tension-Type Headache: Amitriptyline Reduces Clinical Headache-Duration and Experimental Pain Sensitivity but Does Not Alter Pericranial Muscle Activity Readings." *Pain* 59 (1994): 241-9.

Headache Classification Subcommittee of the International Headache Society. "The International Classification of Headache Disorders: 2nd Edition (ICHD-II)." http://ihs-classification.org

Millea, Paul J., J.J. Brodie. "Tension-Type Headache." *American Family Physician* 66, no. 5 (2002): 797-805. http://www.aafp.org/afp/2002/0901/p797.html

Mongini, Franco. *Headaches and Facial Pain*. Stuttgart. Publisher Thieme, 1999.

Moraska, A., and C. Chandler. "Changes in Clinical Parameters in Patients with Tension-Type Headache Following Massage Therapy: A Pilot Study." *Journal of Manual & Manipulative Therapy* 16, no. 2 (2008): 106–12.

National Institute of Neurological Disorders and Stroke, National Institutes of Health. "Headache: Hope Through Research." Publication No. 09-158, 2009. http://www.ninds.nih.gov/disorders/headache/detail_headache.htm

Oguzhanoglu, A., T. Sahiner, T. Kurt, and O. Akalin. "Use of Amitriptyline and Fluoxetine in Prophylaxis of Migraine and Tension-Type Headaches." *Cephalalgia* 19 (1999): 531–2.

Peterson, Cynthia. *The TMJ Healing Plan: Ten Steps to Relieving Headaches, Neck Pain and Jaw Disorders.* Alameda, CA: Hunter House, 2010: 185.

Puustjärvi, K., O. Airaksinen, and P.J. Pöntinen. "The Effects of Massage in Patients with Chronic Tension Headache." *Acupuncture and Electro-Therapeutics Research* 15, no. 2 (1990): 159–62.

Quinn, C., C. Chandler, and A. Moraska. "Massage Therapy and Frequency of Chronic Tension Headaches." *American Journal of Public Health* 92, no. 10 (2002): 1657–61.

Reeves, Alexander G., and R.S. Swenson. "Disorders of the Nervous System: A Primer." Part 2, Chapter 18. 2008. http://www.dartmouth.edu/~dons/part_2/chapter_18.html

Schmidt, M., C. Christiansen, F. Mehnert, K. Rothman, & T. Sørensen. *Non-Steroidal Anti-Inflammatory Drug Use and Risk of Atrial Fibrillation or Flutter: Population Based Case-Control Study.* BMJ Publishing Group. *BMJ* 343 (2011): d3450. http://www.bmj.com/content/343/bmj.d3450

University of Maryland Medical Center. "Tension Headache." http://www.umm.edu/altmed/articles/tension-headache-000074.htm

von Stülpnagel, C., P. Reilich, A. Straube, J. Schäfer, A. Blaschek, S.H. Lee, W. Müller-Felber, V. Henschel, U. Mansmann, and F. Heinen, F. "Myofascial Trigger Points in Children with Tension-Type Headache: A New Diagnostic and Therapeutic Option." *Journal of Child Neurology* 24, no. 4 (2009): 406–9.

Werner, R. *Massage Therapist's Guide to Pathology.* 4th ed. Philadelphia: Lippincott Williams & Wilkins, 2009.

Chapter 7: Migraine Headache Disorders

American Academy of Neurology. "Giving Aspirin Via IV Is Safe and Effective For Severe Headache, Study Finds." *Science Daily.* September 21, 2010. http://www.sciencedaily.com/releases/2010/09/100920172625.htm

American Migraine Foundation. http://www.americanmigrainefoundation.org/whatismigraine.aspx

Aurora, S., M. Gawel, J. Brandes, S. Pokta, and A. Van-Denburgh for the Botox North American Episodic Migraine Study Group. "Botulinum Toxin Type A Prophylactic Treatment of Episodic Migraine: A Randomized, Double-Blind, Placebo-Controlled Exploratory Study." *Headache* 47, no. 4 (2007): 486-99.

Benson, Aaron. "Migraine-Associated Vertigo Overview of Migraines." Medscape Reference. http://emedicine.medscape.com/article/884136-overview

Bigal, M., and A. Krymchantowski. "Emerging Drugs for Migraine Prophylaxis and Treatment." *Medscape General Medicine* 8, no. 2 (2006): 31.

Bigal, M., S. Serrano, D. Buse, A. Scher, W. Stewart, and R. Lipton. "Acute Migraine Medications and Evolution from Episodic to Chronic Migraine: A Longitudinal Population-Based Study." *Headache* 48, no. 8 (2008): 1157-68.

Bigal, M.E., and R.B. Lipton. "Modifiable Risk Factors for Migraine Progression [Review]." *Headache* 46, no. 9 (2006): 1334-43.

Boyer, E.W., and M. Shannon. "The Serotonin Syndrome." *New England Journal of Medicine* 352, no. 11 (2005): 1112-20.

Burstein, R., B. Collins, and M. Jakubowski. "Defeating Migraine Pain with Triptans: A Race Against the Development of Cutaneous Allodynia." *Annals of Neurology* 55, no. 1 (2004): 19-26.

Cady, R., J. Goldstein, R. Nett, R. Mitchell, and R. Browning. "A Double-Blind Placebo-Controlled Pilot Study of Sublingual Feverfew and Ginger (Lipigesic™) in the Treatment of Migraine." *Headache* 51, no. 7 (2011): 1078-86.

Charles, E., and M.D. Argoff. "Using Botulinum Toxin for Headache and Pain." *Medscape Nurses News.* July 2, 2011. http://www.medscape.com/viewarticle/736572

Chu, L.F., D.J. Clark, and M.S. Angst. "Opioid Tolerance and Hyperalgesia in Chronic Pain Patients After One Month of Oral Morphine Therapy: A Preliminary Prospective Study." *Journal of Pain* 7, no. 1 (2006): 43-8.

Cleveland Clinic. "Diseases & Conditions." Patent foramen ovale. http://my.clevelandclinic.org/heart/disorders/congenital/pfo.aspx

Connor, J.G. "Headaches & Migraines." 2010. http://www.compassionateacupuncture.com/Headaches%20&%20Migraines.htm

Diamond, S., M.E. Bigal, S. Silberstein, E. Loder, M. Reed, and R.B. Lipton. "Patterns of Diagnosis and Acute Preventive Treatment for Migraine in the United States: Results from the American Migraine Prevalence and Prevention Study." *Headache* 47 (2007): 355-63.

Dodick, D., R. Lipton, V. Martin, V. Papademetriou, W. Rosamond, A. MaassenVanDenBrink, et al. "Triptan Cardiovascular Safety Expert Panel. Consensus Statement: Cardiovascular Safety Profile of Triptans

(5-HT Agonists) in the Acute Treatment of Migraine." *Headache* 44, no. 5 (2004): 414-25.

Evans, R., and F. Taylor. "'Natural' or Alternative Medications for Migraine Prevention." *Headache* 46, no. 6 (2006): 1012-18.

FDA Public Health Advisory. "Combined Use of 5-Hydroxytryptamine Receptor Agonists (Triptans), Selective Serotonin Reuptake Inhibitors (SSRIs) or Selective Serotonin/Norepinephrine Reuptake Inhibitors (SNRIs)." Created July 19, 2006.

Fife, Terry. "Migraine Associated Vertigo: A Common but Difficult-to-Define Disorder." *Practical Neurology.* 2009. http://bmctoday.net/practicalneu rology/2009/09/article.asp?f=PN0909_02.php

Gandey, Allison. "Botulinum Neurotoxin Reduces Headache Duration." *Medscape Nurses News.* June 25, 2010. http://www.medscape.com/ viewarticle/724237

Headache Classification Subcommittee of the International Headache Society. "The International Classification of Headache Disorders." *Cephalalgia* 24, no. 1 (2004): 9-160.

Ho, T., A. Rodgers , and M. Bigal. "Impact of Recent Prior Opioid Use on Rizatriptan Efficacy. A Post Hoc Pooled Analysis." *Headache* 49, no. 3 (2009): 395-403.

Lassen, L., V. Jacobsen, P. Haderslev, B. Sperling, H.K. Iversen, J. Olesen, and P. Tfelt-Hansen. "Involvement of Calcitonin Gene-Related Peptide in Migraine: Regional Cerebral Blood Flow and Blood Flow Velocity in Migraine Patients." *The Journal of Headache and Pain* 9, no. 3 (2008): 151-7.

Lipton, R., and M.M. Bigal. "Epidemiology, Impact, and Risk Factors for Progression." *Headache* 45, Suppl. 1 (2005): S3-S13. http://www.medscape. com/medline/abstract/15833088

Lipton, R., D. Dodick, R. Sadovsky, K. Kolodner, J. Endicott, J. Hettiarachchi, W. Harrison, and ID Migraine Validation Study. "A Self-Administered Screener for Migraine in Primary Care: The ID Migraine Validation Study." *Neurology* 61 (2003): 375-82.

Lipton, R., W. Stewart, J. Sawyer, and J. Edmeads. "Clinical Utility of an Instrument Assessing Migraine Disability: The Migraine Disability Assessment (MIDAS) Questionnaire." *Headache* 41 (2001): 854-61.

Lipton, Richard B., M. Bigal, S. Ashina, et al. on behalf of the American Migraine Prevalence Prevention Advisory Group. "Cutaneous Allodynia in the Migraine Population." *Annals of Neurology* 63, no. 2 (2008): 148-58.

Mancia, G., E. Agabiti-Rosei, E. Ambrosioni, et al. "Hypertension and Migraine Comorbidity: Prevalence and Risk of Cerebrovascular Events. Evidence From a Large, Multicenter, Cross-Sectional Survey in Italy (MIRACLES study)." *Journal of Hypertension* 29 (2011): 309-18.

Mao, J. "Opioid-Induced Abnormal Pain Sensitivity [Review]." *Current Pain and Headache Reports* 10, no. 1 (2006): 67-70.

Marcus, D. *10 Simple Solutions to Migraines: Recognize Triggers, Control Symptoms, and Reclaim You Life.* Page 3. Oakland, CA: New Harbinger Publications, 2006.

Marcus, D.A. "Treatment of Status Migrainosus." *Expert Opinion on Pharmacotherapy* 2, no. 4 (2001): 549-55.

"Migraine May Double Risk of Heart Attack." From *Science Daily.* February 10, 2010. http://www.sciencedaily.com/releases/2010/02/100210161732.htm

Moskowitz, M.A., K. Nozaki, and R.P. Kraig. "Neocortical Spreading Depression Provokes the Expression of C-Fos Protein-Like Immunoreactivity Within Trigeminal Nucleus Caudalis Via Trigeminovascular Mechanisms." *Journal of Neuroscience* 13 (1993): 1167-77.

Nainggolan, Lisa. "Migraine Could Be Risk Factor for Stroke." June 20, 2011. http://www.theheart.org/article/1241313.do

National Headache Foundation. "Women's Issues in Migraine." 2003.

National Institute of Neurological Disorders and Stroke, National Institutes of Health. "NINDS Migraine Information Page." http://www.ninds.nih.gov/disorders/migraine/migraine.htm

Pappagallo, Marco. *The Neurological Basis of Pain.* New York: McGraw-Hill, Medical Publishing Division, 2005.

Pringsheim, T, W.J. Davenport, and W. Becker. "Prophylaxis of Migraine Headache." *Canadian Medical Association Journal* 182, no. 7 (2010): E269-E76.

Schulman, E., M. Levin, and A. Lake. *Refractory Migraine: Mechanisms and Management.* New York: Oxford University Press, 2010: 47-8.

Shevel, E. "The Extracranial Vascular Theory of Migraine: Evidence Supporting Wolff's Theory that the Extracranial Vasculature is a Source of Pain in Migraine." *Headache* 51, no. 3 (2011): 409-17. Blackwell Publishing. http://www.medscape.com/viewarticle/738527_3

University of Rochester Medical Center. "Mice with a Migraine Show Signs of Brain Damage. Effect on Brain Resembles That From a Mini-Stroke." 2007. http://www.urmc.rochester.edu/news/story/index.cfm?id=1450

Varkey, E., A. Cider, J. Carlsson, and M. Linde. "Exercise as Migraine Prophylaxis: A Randomized Study Using Relaxation and Topiramate as Controls." *Cephalalgia* 31, no. 14 (2011): 1428-38.

Weatherall, M., A. Telzerow, E. Cittadini, H. Kaube, and P.J. Goadsby. "Intravenous Aspirin (lysine acetylsalicylate) in the Inpatient Management of Headache." *Neurology* 75, no. 12 (2010): 1098-103.

Wiley-Blackwell. "Exercise Program Reduces Migraine Suffering." *ScienceDaily.* 2009. http://www.sciencedaily.com/releases/2009/03/090326141557.htm. The study is published in *Headache: The Journal of Head and Face Pain.*

Womenshealth.com. "Migraine Headaches and Patent Foramen Ovale (PFO)." http://www.womens-health.com/boards/general/633-migraine-headaches-patent-foramen-ovale-pfo.html

World Health Organization. "Headache Disorders." Fact Sheet No. 277, March 2004. http://www.who.int/mediacentre/factsheets/fs277/en/

Young, W., S. Silberstein, S. Nahas, and M. Marmura. *Jefferson Headache Manual.* New York: Demos Medical Publishing, 2011: 105-7.

Chapter 8: Primary Headaches in Children

Barclay, Laurie. "Red Ear Syndrome in Children May Be Highly Specific for Migraine." From *Medscape Medical News.* January 14, 2011. http://www.medscape.com/viewarticle/735789

Bechtel, Kirsten. "Pediatric Headache in Emergency Medicine." From Medscape Reference. 2010. http://emedicine.medscape.com/article/802158-medication#2

Bigal, M., and M. Arruda. "Migraine in the Pediatric Population—Evolving Concepts: The Attention Brazil Project—Critical Comment and Advances in Understanding." *Headache* 50, no. 7 (2010): 1130-43.

Boehnke, C., U. Reuter, U. Flach, S. Schuh-Hofer, K. Einhäupl, and G. Arnold. "High-Dose Riboflavin Treatment Is Efficacious in Migraine Prophylaxis: An Open Study in a Tertiary Care Centre." *European Journal of Neurology* 11, no. 7 (2004): 475-77.

Boles, R., M. Lovett-Barr, A. Preston, B.U. Li, and K. Adams. "Treatment of Cyclic Vomiting Syndrome with Co-Enzyme Q10 and Amitriptyline, a Retrospective Study." *Biomed Central* 10 (2010): 10.

Boles, R., A. Powers, and K. Adams. "Cyclic Vomiting Syndrome Plus." *Journal of Child Neurology* 21, no. 3: 182-88.

Boles, R., E. Zaki, T. Lavenbarg, R. Hejazi, P. Foran, J. Freeborn, S. Trilokekar, and R. McCallum. "Are Pediatric and Adult-Onset Cyclic Vomiting Syndrome (CVS) Biologically Different Conditions? Relationship of Adult-Onset CVS With the Migraine and Pediatric CVS-Associated Common Mtdna Polymorphisms 16519T and 3010A." *Neurogastroenterology and Motility* 21, no. 9 (2009): e936-e72.

Cleveland Clinic. "Tension-type Headaches in Children and Adolescents Described." http://my.clevelandclinic.org/disorders/headaches/hic_tension-type_headaches_in_children_and_adolescents.aspx

Fendrich, K., M. Venneman, V. Pfaffenrath, S. Evers, A. May, K. Berger, and W. Hoffmann. "Headache Prevalence Among Adolescents—The German DMKG Headache Study." *Cephalgia* 27 (2007): 347-54.

Headache Classification Subcommittee of the International Headache Society. "The International Classification of Headache Disorders." *Cephalalgia* 24, Suppl. 1 (2004): 9-160.

Headache Classification Subcommittee of the International Headache Society. "The International Classification of Headache Disorders: 2nd Edition (ICHD-II)." http://ihs-classification.org

International Headache Society. "The International Classification of Headache Disorders (ICHD-2)." 1.3.2. Abdominal Migraine.

International Headache Society. "The International Classification of Headache Disorders (ICHD-II)." 1.3.1. Cyclical Vomiting Syndrome.

Lenaerts, M. "Ophthalmologic Manifestations of Pediatric Headache." From Medscape References. 2010. http://emedicine.medscape.com/article/1214702-overview

Lewis, D., P. Winner, A. Hershey, W.W. Wasiewski, and Adolescent Migraine Steering Committee. "Zolmitriptan 5 Mg Nasal Spray for Adolescent Migraine." *Pediatric* 120 (2007): 390–96.

Li, B., F. Lefevre, G. Chelimsky, et al. "North American Society for Pediatric Gastroenterology, Hepatology, and Nutrition Consensus Statement on the Diagnosis and Management of Cyclic Vomiting Syndrome." *Journal of Pediatric Gastroenterology and Nutrition* 47, no. 3 (2008): 379–93.

Lopez, Ivan. "Pediatric Headache." From Medscape References. 2011. http://emedicine.medscape.com/article/1179166-overview

Lu, S., L. Fuh, K. Juang, and S. Wang. "A Student Population-Based Study in Taiwan." *Cephalgia* 20 (2000): 479–85.

McDonald, S., A. Hershey, and E. Pearlman. "Long-Term Evaluation of Sumatriptan and Naproxen Sodium for the Acute Treatment of Migraine in Adolescents." *Headache* 51, no. 9 (2011): 1374–87.

Millichap, J., and M. Yee. "The Diet Factor in Pediatric and Adolescent Migraine." *Pediatric Neurology* 28, no. 1 (2003): 9–15.

Mitchell, A. "Childhood Migraine Variants." From Medscape Reference. 2011. http://emedicine.medscape.com/article/1178141-overview

National Digestive Diseases Information Clearinghouse. *Cyclic Vomiting Syndrome.* NIH Publication No. 09-4548. Bethesda, MD: National Institute of Diabetes and Digestive and Kidney Diseases, 2008.

Pareek, N., D. Fleisher, and T. Abell. "Cyclic Vomiting Syndrome: What a Gastroenterologist Needs to Know." *The American Journal of Gastroenterology* 102, no. 12 (2007): 2832–40.

Popovich, D., D. Schentrup, and A. McAlhany. "Recognizing and Diagnosing Abdominal Migraines: Diagnosis." *Journal of Pediatric Health Care* 24, no. 6 (2010): 372–7.

Rho Y, H. Chung, E. Suh, K.H. Lee, B.L. Eun, S.O. Nam, W.S. Kim, S.H. Eun, and Y.O. Kim. "The Role of Neuroimaging in Children and Adolescents with Recurrent Headaches." *Medscape Nurses News* 51, no. 3 (2011): 403–8.

Robert, Teri. "What Is Hemiplegic Migraine?" From About.com. 2004. http://headaches.about.com/od/migrainediseas1/a/hemiplegic_mig.htm

Van Calcar, S., C. Harding, and J. Wolff. "L-Carnitine Administration Reduces Number Of Episodes in Cyclic Vomiting Syndrome." *Clinical Pediatrics* 41, no. 3 (2002): 171–74.

Chapter 9: Headaches in Women Through the Lifespan

Barclay, L. "NSAID Use in Early Pregnancy Increases Risk for Miscarriage." Medscape Nurses Education. 2011. http://www.medscape.org/viewarticle/749311

De Leo, V., V. Scolaro, M. Musacchio, A. Di Sabatino, G. Morgante, and A. Cianci. "Combined Oral Contraceptives in Women With Menstrual Migraine Without Aura." *Fertility and Sterility* 96, no. 4 (2011): 917-20.

Duong, S., P. Bozzo, H. Nordeng, and A. Einarson. "Safety of Triptans for Migraine Headaches During Pregnancy and Breastfeeding." *Canadian Family Physician* 56, no. 6 (2010): 537-9.

FDA Information for Healthcare Professionals. "Risk of Neural Tube Birth Defects Following Prenatal Exposure to Valproate." 2009. http://www.fda.gov/Drugs/DrugSafety/PostmarketDrugSafetyInformationforPatientsandProviders/DrugSafetyInformationforHeathcareProfessionals/ucm192649.htm

FDA News Release. "Risk of Oral Birth Defects in Children Born to Mothers Taking Topiramate." 2011. http://www.fda.gov/NewsEvents/Newsroom/PressAnnouncements/ucm245594.htm

FDA Questions and Answers. "Risk of Oral Clefts in Infants Born to Mothers Taking Topamax." 2011. http://www.fda.gov/Drugs/DrugSafety/ucm245470.htm

FDA Safety Information and Adverse Event Reporting Program. "Depakote (divalproex sodium) Delayed Release Tablets, Depakote ER (divalproex sodium) Extended Release Tablets, Depakote (divalproex sodium) Sprinkle Capsules." 2009. http://www.fda.gov/Safety/MedWatch/SafetyInformation/Safety-RelatedDrugLabelingChanges/ucm153869.htm

Foley, M. "New Information on the Triptans in Pregnancy." About.com Guide. 2009. http://headaches.about.com/b/2009/11/25/triptans_in_pregnancy.htm

Harms, Roger. "What Can I Do About Headaches During Pregnancy? I'd Rather Not Take Medication." http://www.mayoclinic.com/health/headaches-during-pregnancy/AN01870

Headache Classification Subcommittee of the International Headache Society. "The International Classification of Headache Disorders: 2nd Edition." *Cephalalgia* 24, Suppl. 1 (2004): 9-160.

Hernandez-Diaz, S., R. Mittendorf, and L.B. Holmes. "Comparative Safety of Topiramate During Pregnancy." From Massachusetts General Hospital

Antiepileptic Drug Pregnancy Registry. 2010. http://www.aedpregnan
cyregistry.org/

Loder, E., and D. Marcus. *Migraine in Women.* Ontario: BC Decker, 2004.

MacArthur, Alison. "Differential Diagnosis of Postpartum Headaches."
Revista Mexicana de Anestesologia, Conferencias Magistrales 32,
Suplemento. 1 (2009): S16-S23. http://www.medigraphic.com/pdfs/rma/
cma-2009/cmas091c.pdf

Marcus, Dawn. "Management of Chronic Headache During Pregnancy."
Published in ACHE Newsletter. http://www.dawnmarcusmd.com/lib/
migrainepregnancy.pdf

Mayo Clinic Staff. "Headaches and Hormones: What's the Connection?"
http://www.mayoclinic.com/health/headaches/HE00003

Mayo Clinic Staff. *Mayo Clinic Guide to a Healthy Pregnancy.* Roger Harms,
Editor in Chief. Pymble, NSW: Harper-Collins ebooks.

"Merck Manual Home Health Handbook." *Drug Use During Pregnancy.* http://
www.merckmanuals.com/home/womens_health_issues/drug_use_during_
pregnancy/drug_use_during_pregnancy.html

Pregnancy-Baby-Care.com. "Postpartum Headaches: Conditions, Causes &
Treatment for Postpartum Headaches." http://www.pregnancy-baby-care.
com/postpartum-depression/postpartum-headaches.html

Rasmussen, B. "Migraine and Tension-Type Headache in the General
Population: Precipitating Factors, Female Hormones, Sleep Pattern and
Relation to Lifestyle." *Pain* 53 (1993): 65-72.

Rasmussen, B., R. Jensen, M. Schroll, and J. Olesen. "Epidemiology of
Headache in a General Population-A Prevalence Study." *Journal of Clinical
Epidemiology* 44 (1991): 1147-57.

Rasmussen, B., and J. Olesen. "Migraine with Aura and Migraine Without
Aura: An Epidemiological Study." *Cephalalgia* 12 (1992): 221-28.

Robbins, L., and S. Lang. *Headache Help: A Complete Guide to Understanding
Headaches and the Medications That Relieve Them—Fully Revised and
Updated.* Revised Updated Edition. Mariner Books, 2000.

Russell, M., B. Rasmussen, K. Fenger, and J. Olesen. "Migraine Without Aura
and Migraine with Aura are Distinct Clinical Entities: A Study of Four
Hundred and Eighty-Four Male and Female Migraineurs from the General
Population." *Cephalalgia* 16 (1996): 239-45.

Russell, M., B. Rasmussen, P. Thorvaldsen, and J. Olesen. "Prevalence and Sex
Ratio of the Subtypes of Migraine." *International Journal of Epidemiology*
24 (1995): 612-18.

Russell, Michael Bjørn. "Genetics of Menstrual Migraine: The Epidemiological
Evidence." *Current Pain and Headache Reports* 14, no. 5 (2010): 385-88.

Silberstein, S., and G. Merriam. "Estrogens, Progestins, and Headache."
Neurology 41 (1992): 786-93.

Soldin, O., J. Dahlin, and D. O'Mara. "Triptans in Pregnancy." *Therapeutic Drug Monitoring* 30, no. 1 (2008): 5-9. http://journals.lww.com/drug-monitoring/Abstract/2008/02000/Triptans_in_Pregnancy.2.aspx

Somerville, B. "Estrogen-Withdrawal Migraine. I. Duration of Exposure Required and Attempted Prophylaxis by Premenstrual Estrogen Administration." *Neurology* 25 (1975): 239-44. [PubMed]

Somerville, B. "Estrogen-Withdrawal Migraine. II. Attempted Prophylaxis By Continuous Estradiol Administration." *Neurology* 25 (1975): 245-50.

Somerville, B. "The Role of Estradiol Withdrawal in the Etiology of Menstrual Migraine." *Neurology* 22 (1972): 355-65.

Somerville, B. "The Role of Progesterone in Menstrual Migraine." *Neurology* 21 (1971): 853-59.

Stella, C., C. Jodicke, and H. How. "Postpartum Headache: Is Your Work-Up Complete?" *American Journal of Obstetrics and Gynecology* 196, no. 4 (2007): 318.e1-7.

Chapter 10: Chronic Daily Headaches

Ailani, J. "Chronic Tension-Type Headache." *Current Pain And Headache Reports* 13, no. 6 (2009): 479-83.

Bigal, M., and R. Lipton. "Obesity is a Risk Factor for Transformed Migraine but not Chronic Tension-Type Headache." *Neurology* 67, no. 2 (2006): 252-57.

Couch, J., R. Lipton, W. Stewart, and A. Scher. "Head or Neck Injury Increases the Risk of Chronic Daily Headache: A Population-Based Study." *Neurology* 69, no. 11 (2007): 1169-77.

De Leeuw, R., J. Schmidt, and C. Carlson. "Traumatic Stressors and Post-Traumatic Stress Disorder Symptoms in Headache Patients." *Headache* 45, no. 10 (2005): 1365-74.

Dodick, D.W. "Clinical Practice. Chronic Daily Headache." *New England Journal of Medicine* 354, no. 2 (2006): 158-65.

Headache Classification Subcommittee of the International Headache Society. "The International Classification of Headache Disorders: 2nd Edition." *Cephalalgia* 24, Suppl. 1 (2004): 9-160.

Katsarava, Z., S. Schneeweiss, T. Kurth, U. Kroener, G. Fritsche, A. Eikermann, H.C. Diener, and V. Limmroth. "Incidence and Predictors for Chronicity of Headache in Patients with Episodic Migraine." *Neurology* 62, no. 5 (2004): 788-90.

Lake, A. "Chronic Daily Headache: The Role of the Epidural Blood Patch." *The Internet Journal of Pain, Symptom Control and Palliative Care* 8, no. 1 (2010): 77-80.

Loder, E., and D. Biondi. "Use of Botulinum Toxins for Chronic Headaches: A Focused Review." *Clinical Journal of Pain* 18, no. 6 (2002): S169-76.

Mayo Clinic Staff. "Chronic Daily Headache: Alternative Medicine." http://www.Mayoclinic.Com/Health/Chronic-Daily-Headaches/DS00646/DSECTION=Alternative-Medicine

Scher, A., R. Lipton, and W. Stewart. "Caffeine as a Risk Factor for Chronic Daily Headache: A Population-Based Study." *Neurology* 63, no. 11 (2004): 2022-27.

Scher, A., R. Lipton, and W. Stewart. "Habitual Snoring as a Risk Factor for Chronic Daily Headache." *Neurology* 60, no. 8 (2003): 1366.

Scher, A., R. Lipton, and W. Stewart. "The Comorbidity of Headache with Other Pain Syndromes." *Headache* 46, no. 9 (2006): 1416-23.

Scher, A., L. Midgette, and R. Lipton. "Risk Factors for Headache Chronification: Modifiable Risk Factors for CDH." *Headache* 48, no. 1 (2008): 16-25.

Scher, A., W. Stewart, J. Ricci, and R. Lipton. "Factors Associated with the Onset and Remission of Chronic Daily Headache in a Population-Based Study." *Pain* 106, no. 1-2 (2003): 81-9.

Silberstein, S. "Chronic Daily Headache." *Journal of the American Osteopathic Association* 105, no. 4, (2005): 23S-9S.

Silberstein, S., and D. Liu. "Drug Overuse and Rebound Headache." *Current Pain and Headache Reports* 6, no. 3 (2002): 240-47.

Stovner, L., K. Hagen, R. Jensen, Z. Katsarava, R. Lipton, A. Scher, T. Steiner, and J.A. Zwart. "The Global Burden of Headache: A Documentation of Headache Prevalence and Disability Worldwide." *Cephalalgia* 27, no. 3 (2007): 193-210.

Wiendels, N., A. Neven, F. Rosendaal, P. Spinhoven, F.G. Zitman, W.J. Assendelft, and M.D. Ferrari. "Chronic Frequent Headache in the General Population: Prevalence and Associated Factors." *Cephalalgia* 26, no. 12 (2006): 1434-42.

World Health Organization fact sheet N 277. "Headache Disorders." 2004. http://www.who.int/mediacentre/factsheets/fs277/en/

Chapter 11: Primary Stabbing Headache

Dodick, D. "Indomethacin-Responsive Headache Syndromes." *Current Pain and Headache Report* 8, no. 1 (2004): 19-26. http://www.ncbi.nlm.nih.gov/pubmed/14731379

Headache Classification Subcommittee of the International Headache Society. "The International Classification of Headache Disorders: 2nd Edition (ICHD-II)." http://ihs-classification.org

Loewen, A., M. Hudon, and M. Hill. "Thunderclap Headache and Reversible Segmental Cerebral Vasoconstriction Associated With Use of

Oxymetazoline Nasal Spray." *Canadian Medical Association Journal* 171, no. 6 (2004): 593–94.

Mayo Clinic. "Indomethacin (Oral Route)." http://www.mayoclinic.com/health/drug-information/DR602195

Mayo Clinic. "Melatonin (N-acetyl-5-methoxytryptamine) Safety." http://www.mayoclinic.com/health/melatonin/NS_patient-melatonin/DSECTION=safety.

National Institute of Neurological Disorders and Stroke. "Headache: Hope Through Research." http://www.ninds.nih.gov/disorders/headache/detail_headache.htm

Peterson, C. "Stabbing Headache or Icepick Headache." http://www.migraine-survival.com/ice-pick-headaches

Raskin, N., and R. Schwartz. "Icepick-Like Pain." *Neurology* 30, no. 2 (1980): 203–5.

Rozen, T.D. "Melatonin as Treatment for Idiopathic Stabbing Headache." *Neurology* 61 (2003): 865–66.

Williams, M. *Health Conditions and Concerns: Headaches: Melatonin Relieves Stabbing Headaches.* Bastyr Center for Natural Health, 2004. http://www.bastyrcenter.org/content/view/435/

Chapter 12: Cluster and Related Headaches

Antonaci, F., A. Pareja, A. Caminero, and O. Sjaastad. "Chronic Paroxysmal Hemicrania and Hemicrania Continua: Lack of Efficacy of Sumatriptan." *Headache* 38, no. 3 (1998): 197–200.

Beck, E., W. Sieber, and R. Trejo. "Management of Cluster Headache." *American Family Physician* 71, no. 4 (2005): 717–24. http://www.aafp.org/afp/2005/0215/p717.html

Blau, J., and H. Engel. "A New Cluster Headache Precipitant: Increased Body Heat." *The Lancet* 354, no. 9183 (1999): 1001–2. Referenced in http://www.webmd.com/migraines-headaches/news/19990916/elevated-body-heat-can-cause-cluster-headaches?page=2

Cassels, C. "Zolmitriptan Nasal Spray May Fill Treatment Void for Cluster Headache." *Medscape Medical News.* 2007. http://www.medscape.com/viewarticle/562087

Cohen, A. "Short-Lasting Unilateral Neuralgiform Headache Attacks with Conjunctival Injection and Tearing." *Cephalalgia* 27 (2007): 824.

Cohen, A., M. Matharu, and P. Goadsby. "Double-Blind Placebo-Controlled Trial of Topiramate in SUNCT." *Cephalalgia* 27 (2007): 758.

Cutrer, M., and M. Moskowitz. "Headaches and Other Head Pain." Healthline.com. http://www.healthline.com/elseviercontent/cecil-headaches-and-other-head-pain/3#ixzz1KP7b1sj4.

Etemadifar, M., A. Maghzi, M. Ghasemi, A. Chitsaz, and M. Kaji Esfahani. "Efficacy of Gabapentin in the Treatment of SUNCT Syndrome." *Cephalalgia* 28 (2008): 1339.

Fischera, M., M. Marziniak, I. Gralow, and S. Evers. "The Incidence and Prevalence of Cluster Headache: A Meta-Analysis of Population-Based Studies." *Cephalalgia* 28, no. 6 (2008): 614-8. Epub April 16, 2008. http://www.ncbi.nlm.nih.gov/pubmed/18422717

Goadsby, P.J. "Trigeminal Autonomic Cephalalgias. Pathophysiology and Classification." *Revue Neurologique Société de Neurologie de Paris* 161 (2005): 692.

Headache Classification Subcommittee of the International Headache Society. "The International Classification of Headache Disorders: 2nd Edition." *Cephalalgia* 24, Suppl. 1: 9.

Ikawa, M., N. Imai, and S. Manaka. "A Case of SUNCT Syndrome Responsive to Zonisamide." *Cephalalgia* 31 (2011): 501.

Matharu, M., L. Watkins, and P. Shanahan. "POHo4 Treatment of Medically Intractable SUNCT and SUNA with Occipital Nerve Stimulation." *Journal of Neurology, Neurosurgery and Psychiatry* 81 (2010): e51.

Mayo Clinic Staff. "Cluster Headaches, Overview." http://www.mayoclinic.org/cluster-headaches

National Institute of Neurological Disorders and Stroke. "Headache: Hope Through Research." http://www.ninds.nih.gov/disorders/headache/detail_headache.htm

National Institute of Neurological Disorders and Stroke. "NINDS SUNCT Headache Information Page." http://www.ninds.nih.gov/disorders/sunct/sunct.htm

National Institute of Neurological Disorders and Stroke. "Trigeminal Neuralgia Fact Sheet." http://www.ninds.nih.gov/disorders/trigeminal_neuralgia/detail_trigeminal_neuralgia.htm

Newman, L., R. Spears, and C. Lay. "Hemicrania Continua: A Third Case in Which Attacks Alternate Sides." *Headache* 44, no. 8 (2004): 821-3.

Olesen, J. "The Role of Nitric Oxide (NO) in Migraine, Tension-Type Headache and Cluster Headache." *Pharmacology & Therapeutics* 120, no. 2 (2008): 157-71.

Pareja, J., A. Caminero, E. Franco, J. Casado, J. Pascual, and M. Sánchez del Río. "Dose, Efficacy and Tolerability of Long-Term Indomethacin Treatment of Chronic Paroxysmal Hemicrania and Hemicrania Continua." *Cephalalgia* 21, no. 9 (2001): 906-10.

Peres, M., and S. Silberstein. "Hemicrania Continua Responds to Cyclooxygenase-2 Inhibitors." *Headache* 42, no. 6 (2002): 530-1.

Peres, M., S. Silberstein, S. Nahmias, A.L. Shechter, I. Youssef, and T.D. Rozen, and W.B. Young. "Hemicrania Continua is Not That Rare." *Neurology* 57, no. 6 (2001): 948-51. http://www.neurology.org/content/57/6/948

Pryse-Phillips, W., and J. Murray. "Headache." Healthline.com. http://www.healthline.com/elseviercontent/textbook-headache/5#ixzz1KP8tVQvQ

Schoenen, J. "Cluster Headache." *Advanced Studies in Medicine, Proceedings*, 2001, 446–48. http://www.jhasim.com/files/articlefiles/pdf/Cluster%20Headache.pdf

Sjostrand, C. "Genetic Aspects of Cluster Headache." *Expert Reviews of Neurotherapeutics* 9, no. 3 (2009): 359–68. http://www.clusterattack.com/blog/genetic-aspects-of-cluster-headache/

Chapter 13: Dangerous and Life-Threatening Headaches

Brain Aneurysm Reources. "Incidence Rates of Brain Aneurysms." http://www.brainaneurysm.com/

Brain Cancer Information. "Brain Cancer Studies." http://www.brain-cancer-net.org/brain-cancer-studies.htm

Caserta, M., and A. Flores. "Pharyngitis," in *Principles and Practice of Infectious Diseases*. 7th ed., Chapter 54. Edited by G. Mandell, J. Bennett, and R. Dolin. Philadelphia, PA: Elsevier Churchill Livingstone.

Doheny, K. "Strokes in Children and Young Adults on the Rise." 2011. http://www.m.webmd.com/a-to-z-guides/news/20110901/strokes-in-chldren-and-young-adults-on-the-rise?src=RSS_PUBLIC&utm_source=twitterfeed&utm_medium=twitter

Emedicinehealth. "Brain Aneurysm Overview." http://www.emedicinehealth.com/aneurysm_brain/article_em.htm

Goodwin, James. "Medscape: Drugs, Diseases and Procedures." *Pseudotumor Cerebri Follow-Up.* http://emedicine.medscape.com/article/1143167-followup

Hain, T. "Acoustic Neuroma." 2011. http://www.dizziness-and-balance.com/disorders/tumors/acoustic_neuroma.htm

Headache Classification Subcommittee of the International Headache Society. "The International Classification of Headache Disorders: 2nd Edition (ICHD-II)." http://ihs-classification.org

Huff, S. *Brain Neoplasms.* Medscape Reference: Drugs, Diseases and Procedures. 2012. http://emedicine.medscape.com/article/779664-overview

Johannsen, E., and K. Kaye. "Epstein-Barr Virus (Infectious Mononucleosis, Epstein-Barr Virus-Associated Malignant Diseases, and Other Diseases)," in *Principles and Practice of Infectious Diseases.* 7th ed., Chapter 139. Edited by G. Mandell, J. Bennett, and R. Dolin. Philadelphia, PA: Elsevier Churchill Livingstone.

Kutz, J. "Medscape: Drugs, Diseases and Procedures." *Acoustic Neuroma Treatment & Management.* http://emedicine.medscape.com/article/882876-treatment#a1128

Mayo Clinic Staff. "Brain Tumor Risk Factors." http://www.mayoclinic.com/health/brain-tumor/DS00281/DSECTION=risk-factors

Mayo Clinic Staff. "Pseudotumor Cerebri: Risk Factors." http://www.mayoclinic.com/health/pseudotumor-cerebri/DS00851/DSECTION=risk-factors

Mayo Clinic Staff. "Stroke Causes Discussed." http://www.mayoclinic.com/health/stroke/DS00150/DSECTION=causes

Medical Symptoms Guide. "Pseudotumor Cerebri Overview and Diagnosis." http://www.pseudotumorcerebri.net/

Mukherjee, B. "Acoustic Neuroma Symptoms." 2010. http://www.buzzle.com/articles/acoustic-neuroma-symptoms.html

No authors listed. "The Epidemiology of Headache Among Children With Brain Tumor. Headache in Children with Brain Tumors. The Childhood Brain Tumor Consortium." *Journal of Neurooncology* 10, no. 1 (1991): 31-46.

Peterson, Christina. "What do Brain Tumor Headaches Feel Like? Find Reassurance." http://www.migrainesurvival.com/what-do-brain-tumor-headaches-feel-like-find-reassurance

Reeves, A., and R. Swenson. *Disorders of the Nervous System: A Primer.* Chapter 18. Dartmouth Medical School. http://www.dartmouth.edu/~dons/part_2/chapter_18.html

Ryzenman, J., M. Pensak, and J. Tew. "Headache: A Quality of Life Analysis in a Cohort of 1,657 Patients Undergoing Acoustic Neuroma Surgery, Results from the Acoustic Neuroma Association." *Laryngoscope* 115, no. 4 (2005): 703-11.

Suwanwela, N., K. Phanthumchinda, and S. Kaoropthum. "Headache in Brain Tumor: A Cross-Sectional Study." *Headache: The Journal of Head and Face Pain* 34, no. 7 (1994): 435-38.

University of Pittsburgh Medical Center. "Conditions and Treatments; Pseudotumor Cerebri." http://brainsurgery.upmc.com/conditions-and-treatments/pseudotumor-cerebri.aspx

Chapter 14: Headaches Related to Head Injury

Associated Press. "360k US Troops Suffer Brain Injuries—As Many as 20% of War Vets Have Had Concussions or Worse." 2009. http://www.newser.com/story/52426/360k-us-troops-suffer-brain-injuries.html

Associated Press. "Military Testing Every Returning Soldier for Brain Injuries." *Fox News.* 2009. http://www.foxnews.com/story/0,2933,513581,00.html

Bindera, L. "Persisting Symptoms After Mild Head Injury: A Review of the Postconcussive Syndrome." *Journal of Clinical and Experimental Neuropsychology* 8, no. 4 (1986): 323-46. http://www.ncbi.nlm.nih.gov/pubmed/3091631

Bonthius, D., and A. Lee. "Patient information: Headache in Children." http://www.uptodate.com/contents/patient-information-headache-in-children-beyond-the-basics?source=search_result&search=patient+information+headache+in+children&selectedTitle=1~150

Centers for Disease Control, National Center for Injury Prevention and Control. "Heads Up: Preventing Brain Injuries." http://www.cdc.gov/ncipc/pub-res/tbi_toolkit/patients/preventing.htm

Crippen, D. Head. *Trauma Treatment & Management.* Medscape Reference: Drugs, Diseases & Procedures. 2011. http://emedicine.medscape.com/article/433855-treatment

Edes, G. "Corey Koskie's Clear Head." *Yahoo! Sports.* 2009. http://sports.yahoo.com/mlb/news?slug=ge-koskie022409

Evans, R. *Mild Closed Head Injury and Headache.* American Headache Society. http://www.achenet.org/resources/mild_closed_head_injury_and_headache/

Figueroa, X., and T. Love. "Traumatic Brain Injuries and the Potential of Hyperbaric Oxygen Therapy." http://restorix.com/WP_TBI

Gargollo, P., and A. Lipson. "Brain Trauma, Concussion and Coma From The Dana Guide to Brain Health." 2007. http://www.dana.org/news/brain-health/detail.aspx?id=9790

Haas, D. "Chronic Post-Traumatic Headaches Classified and Compared with Natural Headaches." *Cephalgia* 16, no. 7 (1996): 486-93.

Headache Classification Subcommittee of the International Headache Society. "The International Classification of Headache. Disorders: 2nd Edition." *Cephalalgia* 24, Suppl. 1 (2004): 9-160.

Hendrick, B. "Falls Often to Blame in Traumatic Brain Injury—Traumatic Brain Injuries Kill or Injure Nearly 2 Million People Annually, CDC Report Shows." *WebMD Health News.* 2010. http://www.webmd.com/brain/news/20100318/falls-often-to-blame-in-traumatic-brain-injury.

Hoge, C., D. McGurk, T. Thomas, A.L. Cox, C.C. Engel, and C.A. Castro. "Mild Traumatic Brain Injury in U.S. Soldiers Returning From Iraq." *New England Journal of Medicine* 358, no. 5 (2008): 453-63.

Johnson, G. "Research Finds That Exercise Can Alleviate Post-Concussion Syndrome." Wisconsin Law Blog. 2010. http://wis-injury.com/blog/2010/02/research-finds-that-exercise-can-alleviate-post-concussion-syndrome.html

McDonald, A. "An Interview With Mike Matheny: When Your Head Leads You." *The Hardball Times.* 2010. http://www.hardballtimes.com/main/blog_article/an-interview-with-mike-matheny-when-your-head-leads-you/

National Institute of Neurological Disorders and Stroke. "Traumatic Brain Injury: Hope Through Research." http://www.ninds.nih.gov/disorders/tbi/detail_tbi.htm

PR Newswire. "New Hope and Answers for Returning War Veterans Fighting the Battle Against Post-Traumatic Headache and Migraine." http://www.

prnewswire.com/news-releases/new-hope-and-answers-for-returning-war-veterans-fighting-the-battle-against-post-traumatic-headache-and-migraine-117370148.html

Ravishankar, K., A. Chakravarty, D. Chowdhury, R. Shukla, and S. Singh. "Guidelines on the Diagnosis and the Current Management of Headache and Related Disorders." *Annals of the Indian Academy of Neurology* 14, Suppl. 1 (2011): S40–S59. http://www.ncbi.nlm.nih.gov/pmc/articles/PMC3152170/

Speed, W. *Head Injury and Chronic Headaches.* Health Articles and News Update. http://www.healtharticles.org/head_injury_headaches_071304.html

Thomas, J. "Ex-Steeler Star Hoge Gives Low-Down on Concussions." 2010. http://www.cantonrep.com/sports/x1080710429/Ex-Steeler-star-Hoge-gives-low-down-on-concussions

TraumaticBrainInjury.com. "Understanding Traumatic Brain Injury." 2004. http://www.traumaticbraininjury.com/content/understandingtbi/traumatic-brain-injury-car-accident.html

Weiss, H., B. Stern, and J. Goldberg. "Post-Traumatic Migraine: Chronic Migraine Precipitated by Minor Head or Neck Trauma." *Headache* 31, no. 7 (1991): 451-6.

Yerdon, J. "Marc Savard Speaks Out About Dealing With Post-Concussion Syndrome." ProHockey Talk. 2010. http://prohockeytalk.nbcsports.com/2010/09/25/marc-savard-speaks-out-about-dealing-with-post-concussion-syndrome/

Chapter 15: Inflammatory and Noninfectious Diseases and Headaches

Aaron, L., M. Burke, and D. Buchwald, D. "Overlapping Conditions Among Patients With Chronic Fatigue Syndrome, Fibromyalgia, and Temporomandibular Disorder." *Archives of Internal Medicine* 160 (2000): 221-7.

Ablashi, D., Z. Berneman, C. Lawyer, B. Kramarsky, D.M. Ferguson, and A.L. Komaroff. "Antiviral Activity in Vitro of Kutapressin Against Human Herpesvirus-6." *In Vivo* 8, no. 4 (1994): 581-6.

Bley, T., M. Uhl, J. Carew, M. Markl, D. Schmidt, H.H. Peter, M. Langer, and O. Wieben. "Diagnostic Value of High-Resolution MR Imaging in Giant Cell Arteritis." *American Journal of Neuroradiology* 28, no. 9 (2007): 1722-7.

Brenu, E., M. van Driel, D. Staines, K.J. Ashton, S.B. Ramos, J.Keane, N.G. Klimas and S.M. Marshall-Gradisnik. "Immunological abnormalities as potential biomarkers in Chronic Fatigue Syndrome/Myalgic Encephalomyelitis." *Journal of Translational Medicine* 9 (2011): 81.

Center for Disease Control and Prevention. "Systemic Lupus Erythematosus Defined." http://www.cdc.gov/arthritis/basics/lupus.htm

Chan, C., M. Paine, and J. O'Day. "Steroid Management in Giant Cell Arteritis." *British Journal of Ophthalmology* 85, no. 9 (2001): 1061-4.

De Tommaso, M., A. Federici, C. Serpino, E. Vecchio, G. Franco, M. Sardaro, M. Delussi, and P. Livrea. "Clinical Features of Headache Patients With Fibromyalgia Comorbidity." *Journal of Headache Pain* 12, no. 6 (2011): 629-38.

Duke Center for Human Genetics. "Multiple Sclerosis Discussed." http://www.chg.duke.edu/diseases/ms.html

Fibromyalgia Symptoms. "Headaches and Fibromyalgia Described." http://www.fibromyalgia-symptoms.org/fibromyalgia_chronic_headaches.html

Freeman, H. "Adult Celiac Disease Followed by Onset of Systemic Lupus Erythematosus." *Journal of Clinical Gastroenterology* 42, no. 3 (2008): 252-5.

Gee, J.R., J. Chang, A.B. Dublin, and N. Vijayan. "The Association of Brainstem Lesions With Migraine-Like Headache: An Imaging Study of Multiple Sclerosis." *Headache* 45, no. 6 (2005): 670-7.

Gentile, S., M. Ferrero, G. Vaula, I. Rainero, and L. Pinessi. "Cluster Headache Attacks and Multiple Sclerosis." *J Headache Pain* 8, no. 4 (2007): 245-7.

Help for Headaches. "Fibromyalgia and Chronic Headache Described." http://www.headache-help.org/fibromyalgia-and-chronic-headache

International Painful Bladder Foundation. "Painful Bladder Syndrome/Interstitial Cystitis and Associated Disorders—An Overview." http://www.painful-bladder.org/pbs-ic_ass_dis_introduction.html

Johns Hopkins Vasculitis Center. "Giant Cell Arteritis Described." http://www.hopkinsvasculitis.org/types-vasculitis/giant-cell-arteritis/

Johns Hopkins Lupus Center. "Nervous System and Lupus." http://www.hopkinslupus.org/lupus-info/lupus-affects-body/lupus-nervous-system/

Johns Hopkins Lupus Center. "Signs, Symptoms, and Co-Occuring Conditions of Lupus." http://www.hopkinslupus.org/lupus-info/lupus-signs-symptoms-comorbidities/

Katsiari, C., and M. Vikelis. "Headache in Systemic Lupus Erythematosus vs Multiple Sclerosis: A Prospective Comparative Study." *Headache: The Journal of Head and Face Pain* 51, no. 9 (2011): 1398-407.

Lawrence, R., D. Felson, C. Helmick, et al. "Estimates of the Prevalence of Arthritis and Other Rheumatic Conditions in the United States. Part II." National Arthritis Data Workgroup. *Arthritis and Rheumatism* 58, no. 1 (2007): 26-35.

Levine, S., J.W. Crofts, G.R. Lesser, J. Floberg, and K.M. Welch. "Visual Symptoms Associated with the Presence of a Lupus Anticoagulant." *Ophthalmology* 95 (1988): 686-92.

Living With Chronic Fatigue Syndrome. WordPress.com weblog. October 25, 2010. "Nexavir (Kutapressin) for CFS." http://livingwithchronicfatiguesyndrome.wordpress.com/2010/10/25/nexavir-kutapressin-for-cfs/

Lupus Foundation of America. "How Lupus Affects the Body: Nervous System." 2009. http://www.lupus.org/webmodules/webarticlesnet/templates/new_aboutaffects.aspx?articleid=102&zoneid=17

Lupus Foundation of America. "Lupus Headache Described." http://www.lupus.org/webmodules/webarticlesnet/templates/new_aboutaffects.aspx?a=102&z=0&page=2

Lupus Foundation of America. "Lupus Headaches in Children Described." http://www.lupus.org/webmodules/webarticlesnet/templates/new_research.aspx?articleid=1694&zoneid=3

Lupus Site, The. "Lupus: The Symptoms and Diagnosis." http://www.uklupus.co.uk/fact3.html

Martinez-Lado, L., C. Calviño-Díaz, A. Piñeiro, T. Dierssen, T.R. Vazquez-Rodriguez, J.A. Miranda-Filloy, M.J. Lopez-Diaz, R. Blanco, J. Llorca, and M.A. Gonzalez-Gay. "Relapses and Recurrences in Giant Cell Arteritis: A Population-Based Study of Patients with Biopsy-Proven Disease From Northwestern Spain." *PubMed, Medicine (Baltimore)* 90, no. 3 (2011): 186–93.

Mayo Clinic Staff. "Chronic Fatigue Syndrome Defined." http://www.mayoclinic.com/health/chronic-fatigue-syndrome/DS00395/DSECTION-symptoms

Mitsikostas, Dimos D., Petros P. Sfikakis, and P. Goadsby. "A Meta-Analysis for Headache in Systemic Lupus Erythematosus: The Evidence and the Myth." *Primary Reference: Brain* 127, no. 5 (2004): 1200–9.

MultipleSclerosis.org. "Optic Neurtitis." http://www.mult-sclerosis.org/optic-neuritis.html

National Fibromyalgia Research Association. "Headaches Described." http://www.nfra.net/fibromyalgia-headaches.htm

New York Headache Center. "Magnesium and Headaches Discussed." http://nyheadache.com/index.php?option=com_content&view=article&id=39&Itemid=76

Noonan, C., D. Williamson, J. Henry, R. Indian, S.G. Lynch, J.S. Neuberger, R. Schiffer, J. Trottier, L. Wagner, and R.A. Marrie. "The Prevalence of Multiple Sclerosis in 3 US Communities." *Preventing Chronic Disease* 7, no. 1 (2010): A12.

Pigache, P. *Positive Options for Living with Lupus.* Alameda, CA: Hunter House Publishers, 2006: 41, 52, 91.

Pisetsky, D., J. Buyon, and S. Manzi. "Systemic Lupus Erythematosus." From Chapter 17 of the *Primer on the Rheumatic Diseases, Edition 12* by Klippel, Crofford, Stone, Weyand. Atlanta, GA: Arthritis Foundation, 2001.

Reeves, A., and R. Swenson. *Disorders of the Nervous System: A Primer.* Chapter 18. Dartmouth Medical School. http://www.dartmouth.edu/~dons/part_2/chapter_18.html

Rosenfeld, E., B. Salimi, M. O'Gorman, C. Lawyer, and B.Z. Katz. "Potential in Vitro Activity of Kutapressin Against Epstein-Barr Virus." *In Vivo* 10, no. 3 (1996): 313-8. http://www.webmd.com/fibromyalgia/features/living-with-fibromyalgia-and-chronic-fatigue

Rus, V., A. Hajeer, and M. Hochberg. "Systemic Lupus Erythematosus." From Chapter 7 of *Epidemiology of the Rheumatic Disease, 2nd edition* by AJ Silman and MC Hochberg editors. New York, NY: Oxford University Press, 2001.

Savella. http://www.savella.com/index.aspx

Shin, C., L. Bateman, R. Schlaberg, A.M. Bunker, C.J. Leonard, R.W. Hughen, A.R. Light, K.C. Light, and I.R. Singh. "Absence of XMRV and Other MLV-Related Viruses in Patients with Chronic Fatigue Syndrome." *Journal of Virology* 2011 (2011). doi: 10.1128/JVI.00693-11

Skelly, M., and H. Walker. *Alternative Treatments for Fibromyalgia and Chronic Fatigue Syndrome.* 2nd ed. Alameda, CA: Hunter House, 2006.

Smith, J., H. Stock, S. Bingaman, D. Mauger, M. Rogosnitzky, and I.S. Zagon. "Low-Dose Naltrexone Therapy Improves Active Crohn's Disease." *American Journal of Gastroenterology* 102, no. 4 (2007): 820-8.

Wallace, Daniel J. "Heady Connections: The Nervous System and Behavioral Changes." *The Lupus Book: A Guide for Patients and Their Families.* 1st ed. New York, NY: Oxford University Press, 1995: 99-115.

Weder-Cisneros, N., J. Téllez-Zenteno, M. Cardiel, M. Guibert-Toledano, J. Cabiedes, A.L. Velásquez-Paz, G. García-Ramos, and C. Cantú. "Prevalence and Factors Associated with Headache in Patients with Systemic Lupus Erythematosus." *Cephalalgia* 24, no. 12 (2004): 1031-44.

Weinberger, J. "Stroke and Migraine." *Current Cardiology Reports* 9, no. 1 (2007): 13-9.

Chapter 16: Headaches and Infectious Diseases

American Academy of Otolaryngology—Head and Surgery. "Sinus Headaches." http://www.entnet.org/HealthInformation/sinusHeadache.cfm

Avitzur, Orly. "Daily Persistent Headache Following Mononucleosis." *Medscape Nurses News.* 2004. http://www.medscape.com/viewarticle/472661

Brad Klein, B., and S. Silberstein, ed. "Headache Associated With AIDS." Originally released August 9, 1994; last updated September 25, 2011; expires September 25, 2014. Medlink Neurology. https://www.medlink.com/medlinkcontent.asp

Brannon, H. "Shingles Complications." http://dermatology.about.com/od/infectionvirus/a/shingles_comp.htm

Centers for Disease Control and Prevention, National Center for Infectious Diseases. "Epstein-Barr Virus and Infectious Mononucleosis." www.cdc.gov/ncidod/diseases/ebv.htm

Centers for Disease Control and Prevention. "Sinus Infection (Sinusitis)." http://www.cdc.gov/getsmart/antibiotic-use/URI/sinus-infection.html

Cooper, D., J. Gold, P. Maclean, B. Donovan, R. Finlayson, T.G. Barnes, H.M. Michelmore, P. Brooke, and R. Penny. "Acute AIDS Retrovirus Infection. Definition of a Clinical Illness Associated With Seroconversion." *Lancet* 1, no. 8428 (1985): 537-40.

Eastern, J. "Herpes Zoster." http://emedicine.medscape.com/article/1132465-overview

Eross, E., D. Dodick, and M. Eross. "The Sinus, Allergy and Migraine Study (SAMS)." *Headache* 47, no. 2 (2007): 213-24.

Evans, R. "New Daily Persistent Headache." *Current Pain and Headache Reports* 7 (2003): 303-7.

Goldstein, J. "Headache and Acquired Immunodeficiency Syndrome." *Neurologic Clinics* 8 (1990): 947-60.

Guo, R., P. Cantery, and E. Ernst. "Herbal Medicines for the Treatment of Rhinosinusitis: A Systematic Review." Sage Journals. 2006. http://oto.sagepub.com/content/135/4/496.abstract

Hope-Simpson, R.E. "The Nature of Herpes Zoster; A Long-Term Study and a New Hypothesis." *Proceedings of the Royal Society of Medicine* 58 (1965): 9-20. http://www.pubmedcentral.nih.gov/articlerender.fcgi?tool=pmcentrez&artid=1898279

Li, D., and T. Rozen. "The Clinical Characteristics of New Daily Persistent Headache." *Cephalalgia* 22 (2002): 66-9.

Mayo Clinic Staff. "Chronic Daily Headaches." http://www.mayoclinic.com/health/chronic-daily-headaches/DS00646

Mayo Clinic Staff. "Sinus Headaches." http://www.mayoclinic.com/health/sinus-headaches/DS00647/DSECTION=prevention

Meltzer, E., D. Hamilos, J. Hadley, et al. "Rhinosinusitis: Establishing Definitions for Clinical Research and Patient Care." *Journal of Allergy and Clinical Immunology* 114, no. 6 Suppl (2004): 155-212.

Michigan Headache and Neurological Institute. "Diagnosis and Treatment of New Daily Persistent Headache." www.mhni.com/faqs_ndph.aspx

Mirsattari, S.M., C. Power, and A. Nath. "Primary Headaches in HIV-Infected Patients in a Neuro-AIDS Clinic. Neuroscience of HIV Infection." *Journal of Neurovirology* 4 (1998): 360. http://gateway.nlm.nih.gov/MeetingAbstracts/ma?f=102237443.html

Moon, J., D. Hospenthal, R. Krause, and M. Wallace. "Herpes Zoster." *Medscape Reference: Drugs, Diseases, and Procedures.* http://emedicine.medscape.com/article/788310-overview

National Institute of Allergy and Infectious Diseases. "Sinusitis." http://www.niaid.nih.gov/topics/sinusitis/Pages/index.aspx

OrganizedWisdom Team. "Sinus Headaches and Alternative Medicine." http://www.organizedwisdom.com/Sinus_Headaches_and_Alternative_Medicine

The University of Maryland Medical Center. "CSF Leak—An Overview." www.umm.edu/ency/article/001068.htm

The University of Maryland Medical Center. "Sinus Headache." http://www.umm.edu/altmed/articles/sinus-headache-000073.htm

Tindall, B., A. Imrie, B. Donovan, R. Penny, and D.A. Cooper. "Primary HIV Infection." In: Sande MA and Volberding PA, editors. *The Medical Management of AIDS*. 3rd ed. Philadelphia: WB Saunders, 1992: 67-86.

U.S. Food and Drug Administration. "Zostavax (Herpes Zoster Vaccine) Questions and Answers." http://www.fda.gov/BiologicsBloodVaccines/Vaccines/QuestionsaboutVaccines/UCM070418

Weil, Andrew. Q & A Library. "Snuffing Out a Sinus Infection." http://www.drweil.com/drw/u/id/QAA326609

Chapter 17: The Future of Headache Care

Bagdy, G., P. Riba, V. Kecskeméti, D. Chase, and G. Juhász. "Headache-Type Adverse Effects of NO Donors: Vasodilation and Beyond." *British Journal of Pharmacology* 160, no. 1 (2010): 20-35. http://www.ncbi.nlm.nih.gov/pmc/articles/PMC2860203/

Brandes, J., R. Cady, F. Freitag, T.R. Smith, P. Chandler, A.W. Fox, L. Linn, and S.J. Farr. "Needle-Free Subcutaneous Sumatriptan (Sumavel Dosepro): Bioequivalence and Ease of Use." *Headache* 49, no. 10 (2009): 1435-44.

Brandes, J., D. Kudrow, S.R. Stark, C.P. O'Carroll, J.U. Adelman, F.J. O'Donnell, W.J. Alexander, S.E. Spruill, P.S. Barrett, and S.E. Lener. "Sumatriptan-Naproxen for Acute Treatment of Migraine: A Randomized Trial." *Journal of the American Medical Association* 297, no. 13 (2007): 1443-54.

Durham, P., and C. Vause. "CNS Drugs: CGRP Receptor Antagonists in the Treatment of Migraine." *CNS Drugs* 24, no. 7 (2010): 539-48. http://www.ncbi.nlm.nih.gov/pmc/articles/PMC3138175/

Goadsby, P., R. Lipton, and M. Ferrari. "Migraine—Current Understanding and Treatment." *New England Journal of Medicine* 346, no. 4 (2002): 257-70. https://secure.muhealth.org/~ed/students/articles/NEJM_346_p257.pdf

Goldstein, J., N. Pugach, and T. Smith. "Acute Anti-Migraine Efficacy and Tolerability of Zelrix, a Novel Iontophoretic Transdermal Patch of Sumatriptan." *Cephalalgia* 29, no. s1 (2009): 20.

Halker, R. *Single-Pulse Transcranial Magnetic Stimulation as a Potential Acute Treatment for Migraine with Aura*. American Migraine Foundation,

January 10, 2011. http://www.americanmigrainefoundation.org/service/news.aspx?CategoryId=1&ArticleId=56

Hauge,A.,M.Asghar,H.Schytz,K.Christensen,andJ.Olesen."EffectsofTonabersat on Migraine With Aura: A Randomised, Double-Blind, Placebo-Controlled Crossover Study." *The Lancet Neurology* 8, no. 8 (2009): 718-23. http://www.thelancet.com/journals/laneur/article/PIIS1474-4422(09)70135-8/abstract

Ho, T., M. Ferrari, and D. Dodick. "Efficacy and Tolerability of MK-0974 (Telcagepant), a New Oral Antagonist of Calcitonin Gene-Related Peptide Receptor, Compared With Zolmitriptan for Acute Migraine: A Randomised, Placebo-Controlled, Parallel-Treatment Trial." *The Lancet* 372, no. 9656 (2008): 2115-23. http://www.thelancet.com/journals/lancet/article/PIIS0140-6736(08)61626-8/fulltext

Hoffmann, J., and P. Goadsby. "New Agents for Acute Treatment of Migraine: CGRP Receptor Antagonists, iNOS Inhibitors." *Current Treatment Options in Neurology* 14, no. 1 (2012): 50-9. http://www.ncbi.nlm.nih.gov/pubmed/22090312

Holland, P., C. Schembri, J. Fredrick, and P. Goadsby. "Transcranial Magnetic Stimulation for the Treatment of Migraine Aura?" *Cephalalgia* 29, no. s1 (2009): 22.

Lassen, L., L. Thomsen, and J. Olesen. "Histamine Induces Migraine Via the H1-Receptor. Support for the NO Hypothesis of Migraine." *Neuroreport* 31 (1995): 1475-9. http://www.ncbi.nlm.nih.gov/pubmed/7579128

Lipton, R., D. Dodick, S. Silberstein, J.R. Saper, S.K. Aurora, S.H. Pearlman, R.E. Fischell, P.L. Ruppel, and P.J. Goadsby. "Single-Pulse Transcranial Magnetic Stimulation for Acute Treatment of Migraine with Aura: A Randomised, Double-Blind, Parallel-Group, Sham-Controlled Trial." *The Lancet Neurology* 9, no. 4 (2010): 373-80. http://www.ncbi.nlm.nih.gov/pubmed/20206581

Lyngberg, A., B. Rasmussen, T. Jorgensen, and R. Jensen"Incidence of Primary Headache: A Danish Epidemiologic Follow-Up Study." *American Journal of Epidemiology* 161 (2005): 1066-73. http://aje.oxfordjournals.org/content/161/11/1066.full.pdf

Monteith, T., and P. Goadsby. "Acute Migraine Therapy: New Drugs and New Approaches." *Current Treatment Options in Neurology* 13, no. 1 (2011): 1-14. http://www.springerlink.com/content/572681472811v253/

Olesen, J. "The Role of Nitric Oxide (NO) in Migraine, Tension-Type Headache and Cluster Headache." *Pharmacology & Therapeutics* 120, no. 2 (2008): 157-71. http://www.ncbi.nlm.nih.gov/pubmed/18789357

Olesen, J., H. Diener, I. Husstedt, P.J. Goadsby, D. Hall, U. Meier, S. Pollentier, L.M. Lesko, and BIBN 4096 BS Clinical Proof of Concept Study Group. "Calcitonin Gene-Related Peptide Receptor Antagonist BIBN 4096 BS for the Acute Treatment of Migraine." *New England*

Journal of Medicine 350, no. 11 (2004): 1104–10. http://www.ncbi.nlm. nih.gov/pubmed/15014183

Olesen, J., P. Tfelt-Hansen, and M. Ashina. "Finding New Drug Targets for the Treatment of Migraine Attacks." *Cephalalgia* 29, no. 9 (2002): 909–20. http://www.ncbi.nlm.nih.gov/pubmed/19250288

Parsons, M., and C. Ganellin. "Histamine and Its Receptors." *British Journal of Pharmacology* 147 (2006): S127–35.

PR Newswire. "MAP Pharmaceuticals Announces Successful Results for LEVADEX™ Thorough QT Trial." 2010. http://www.prnewswire.com/news-releases/map-pharmaceuticals-announces-successful-results-for-levadex-thorough-qt-trial-106876798.html

Ramadan, N., V. Skljarevski, L. Phebus, and K. Johnson. "5-HT1F Receptor Agonists in Acute Migraine Treatment: A Hypothesis." *Cephalalgia* 23, no. 8 (2003): 776–85. http://www.ncbi.nlm.nih.gov/pubmed/14510923

Silberstein, S., S. Kori, S. Tepper, et al. "Efficacy and Tolerability of MAP0004, a Novel Orally Inhaled Therapy in Treating Acute Migraine." *Cephalalgia* 1, no. s1 (2009): 12.

Chapter 18: Coping Measures and Support Strategies

Batiste, L. "How to Determine Whether a Person Has a Disability under the Americans with Disabilities Act Amendments Act (ADAAA)." Job Accommodation Network. *Consultants' Corner* 5, no. 4. http://askjan.org/corner/vol05iss04.htm

Bromberg, J., M. Wood, R. Black, D. Surette, K.L. Zacharoff, and E.J. Chiauzzi. "A Randomized Trial of a Web-Based Intervention to Improve Migraine Self-Management and Coping." *Headache: The Journal of Head and Face Pain* 52, no. 2 (2012): 244–61.

Kurth, T., M. Schürks, G. Logroscino, and J.E. Buring. "Migraine Frequency and Risk of Cardiovascular Disease in Women." *Neurology* 2010, no. 74 (2009): 615–16.

Lee, D. "10 Things You Should Know About Chronic Migraines and Applying for Social Security Disability." Migraine.com Blogs. 2011. http://migraine.com/blog/10-things-you-should-know-about-chronic-migraines-and-applying-for-social-security-disability/

MacClellan, L.R., W. Giles, J. Cole, M. Wozniak, B. Stern, B.D. Mitchell, and S.J. Kittner. "Probable Migraine With Visual Aura and Risk of Ischemic Stroke: The Stroke Prevention in Young Women Study." *Stroke* 38 (2007): 2438–45.

McKay, D. "Disability Benefits—If You Can't Work You May Be Eligible for Government Disability Benefits." About.com Guide. http://careerplanning.about.com/cs/legalissues/a/dis_benefits.htm

National Migraine Association. "MAGNUM's Draft Legislation–Medical & Political Justification–Medical Evaluation Criteria for the Migraine Disease. RE: Disability Evaluation Criteria Under Social Security Parts A & B' Listing of Impairments." http://www.migraines.org/disability/disableg.htm

Robert, T. "Disability: When Migraines Stop You, in the Words of Migraineurs." About.com Guide. 2003. http://headaches.about.com/cs/disability/a/mig_disability.htm

Social Security Online. "Disability Planner: Social Security Protection If You Become Disabled." http://www.ssa.gov/dibplan/index.htm

U.S. Department of Labor, Wage and Hour Division (WHD). "Family and Medical Leave Act." http://www.dol.gov/whd/fmla/

Appendix—
The Weekly Headache
Diary, a Useful Tool

Please use the sample headache diary on the following pages to track your headache symptoms on a weekly basis. Keep this tool close at hand for when a headache strikes, and also take it with you to your doctor's appointments. It will provide your doctor with useful information to consider when planning your care. In the diary tool, you will see "24 HR FOOD & FLUID INTAKE." This refers to all the foods and fluids you have consumed in the 24 hours *leading up* to the development of headache symptoms. Recording this information will allow you to recognize patterns and identify possible headache triggers. Even if you do not experience a headache on a given day, it is still a good idea to track your food and fluid intake, because these may be important factors in headache prevention.

The New England Regional Headache Center website also has a downloadable headache diary form and other tools that you may find useful. See: www.nerhc.org/nss-folder/folder.

Weekly Headache Diary

Dates	Time HA onset	Time HA relief	Any factors contributing to HA?	HA Pain Scale 0-10[a]	Describe HA character	Associated HA symptoms[b]	Disability Scale 1-5[c]	Comfort treatments & effect	Medications taken & effect	Exercise past 24 hours?
SUNDAY										
24 HR INTAKE FOOD & FLUIDS:										
MONDAY										
24 HR INTAKE FOOD & FLUIDS:										
TUESDAY										
24 HR INTAKE FOOD & FLUIDS:										
WEDNESDAY										
24 HR INTAKE FOOD & FLUIDS:										

[a]Rate headache pain on a scale from 0 to 10, with 10 being the worst possible pain.

[b]Such as nausea, vomiting, visual effects, sensitivity to light, sound, or touch?

[c]Rate disability using the following: (1) able to continue working or routine, (2) symptoms interfere with normal work or routine, (3) severely impaired and unable to continue normal work or routine, (4) bed rest required, and (5) medical treatment required by emergency room or doctor.

Dates	Time HA onset	Time HA relief	Any factors contributing to HA?	HA Pain Scale 0–10[a]	Describe HA character	Associated HA symptoms[b]	Disability Scale 1–5[c]	Comfort treatments & effect	Medications taken & effect	Exercise past 24 hours?
THURSDAY										
24 HR INTAKE FOOD & FLUIDS:										
FRIDAY										
24 HR INTAKE FOOD & FLUIDS:										
SATURDAY										
24 HR INTAKE FOOD & FLUIDS:										

[a] Rate headache pain on a scale from 0–10, with 10 being the worst possible pain.

[b] Such as nausea, vomiting, visual effects, sensitivity to light, sound, or touch?

[c] Rate disability using the following: (1) able to continue working or routine, (2) symptoms interfere with normal work or routine, (3) severely impaired and unable to continue normal work or routine, (4) bed rest required, and (5) medical treatment required by emergency room or doctor.

Weekly Notes:

Index